GOVERNING HOSPITALS

Trustees and the
New Accountabilities

Robert M. Cunningham Jr.

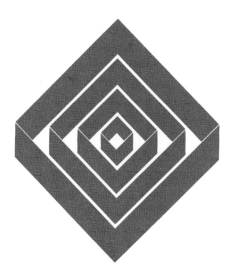

The American Hospital Association
840 North Lake Shore Drive
Chicago, Illinois 60611

Library of Congress Cataloging in Publication Data
Cunningham, Robert Maris, 1909-
  Governing hospitals.

  Includes bibliographical references and index.
  1. Hospitals—Trustees. I. Title. [DNLM:
1. Governing board. 2. Hospital administration.
WX150 0973g]
RA971.C79   658.4'2   75-44127
ISBN 0-87258-182-9

AHA catalog no. 1665
© 1976 by the
American Hospital Association
840 North Lake Shore Drive
Chicago, Illinois 60611

Printed in the U.S.A.
16M-1/76-4822
7M-2/77-5539

Designed by
Claude J. Zajakowski

Printed by
Visual Images Inc.
Waukegan, Illinois

CONTENTS

PREFACE

Years ago, as a fledgling staff member of the Plan for Hospital Care, then a new and in some circles suspect enterprise that has gained weight and respectability over the years and is now known as Blue Cross, I had, among other duties, the assignment of attending meetings of hospital boards of trustees to explain what my employers were up to and answer questions about our solvency, our prospects, and our intentions, usually in that order. In preparing for one of these often intimidating occasions, I usually obtained a copy of the hospital's annual report, which in those pre-public relations days was invariably printed in black ink on white paper and consisted largely of statistical and financial reports and lists of donors whose benefices ranged from bridge tables to buildings. The reports were not what anybody would call fascinating reading, but they gave me the information I wanted—the names of the trustees and the dimensions of the operation. For all their color photographs and high-toned prose, today's annual reports don't tell us much more and aren't that much easier to read.

Then, as now, the lists of trustees commonly included an identifying line with every name. Chairmen and presidents abounded; banks and utilities were the favored pursuits, clearly preferred to merchandise and manufacture. Trustee Smith of Smith, Jones, Parker & Scott was obviously in those days the senior partner of a prestigious law firm; the same designation today might as readily identify a public accountant or management consultant. Today's lists, too, have fewer reverends and more MDs. The presence of a physician among the chairmen and presidents and senior partners in the old days was nearly always an indication of emeritus status on the medical staff, and usually was so stated; the election of an active practicing physician to the board, now a common though still not wholly accepted phenomenon, was regarded as a breach not so much of ethics or good practice as of etiquette, like wearing a sports coat to the office. The lone woman member was the president of the women's, or ladies' (as they were then called), auxiliary. If there was a second woman in the room at board meetings, it was the administrator, or superintendent, and the assembled executives and capitalists listened respectfully when she spoke; she was a nurse and thus a bridge to the mysterious dominions of medicine. The male administrator who was unprotected by either the mystique of the MD or the sanctity of the cloth was at a disadvantage. He was ordinary mortal flesh, and probably not too robust, at that, or he would be out there making his fortune like any other redblooded American. The latter-day administrator is under no such handicap. He was professionally trained for his assignment, for one thing, and can trade flowcharts and data inputs with any banker or management consultant in the boardroom. For another, he knows the ins and outs of all the titles and sections and paragraphs of the new laws, and the regulations pertaining thereto, and these have all but supplanted the cabalistic signs of the operating room and the medical record in their capacity to confound and frustrate the unanointed.

For the most part, details of the hospital board meetings I attended so many years ago have long since been forgotten, but I do recall being surprised at the amount of time trustees would spend examining detailed accounts of income and expense, just as I have been surprised in recent years when trustees have unblinkingly accepted huge increments of expense and approved vast capital undertakings. Unquestionably, the contrast owes more to inflation than to any difference in the performance of trustees. I remember, too, that the chairmen and presidents were interested and courteous in their response to my presentations of the prepayment concept, but their willingness to participate in the new scheme depended on weightier considerations than those adduced by me. Directors of the Plan were all community leaders—fellow chairmen, presidents, and senior partners—and the Plan appeared to offer the possibility, at least, that some of the empty beds might be filled and paid for. The only misgiving that ever came up was that the doctors wouldn't like it, and they didn't. Some of the trustees had already heard that the doctors thought prepayment was a form of, or forerunner to, socialized medicine and didn't want any part of it. This was my clue to argue that, quite on the contrary, voluntary prepayment was the best protection *against* socialized medicine. The argument is still going on, and the facts are not altogether clear, but, if anything, I am less persuaded now than I was then that I was right and the doctors were wrong. For better or worse, however, the trustees were mostly on my side.

In some hospitals then, and a few still, the boardroom and administrator's office were the same domain, and the occupants were all female: the Mother or Sister Superior and a few trusted, and usually silent, assistants. I remember a meeting with one such board, or executive cadre, that comes to mind now whenever I have occasion to report a meeting or conversation concerning the extraordinary complexities of hospital financial operations in the era of "reasonable cost" reimbursement. The Plan for Hospital Care had been operating for several months and, through the type of accounting error that has not been notably diminished by the advent of the computer, had overpaid one of the Sisters' hospitals by several hundred dollars for services rendered to Plan members. The Sisters owed us the money, and I was dispatched to the hospital to convey the glad tidings and make arrangements for settlement of the debt, a task for which I was as ill-prepared then as I was years later to write about the intricacies of the RCCAC* method of stepdown cost finding in Medicare. The theory was that such an occasion was a public relations opportunity, a proposition that fails every test of reason but can still be heard around the ritual campfires of public relations practitioners.

The meeting, with Sister Administrator and Sister Accountant and one or two others whose identity remained uncertain, was not an unqualified success. Given the dismal circumstances and my dim grasp of the accounting process involved, this was scarcely surprising. After toiling through the records, ours and theirs, however, the Sisters were convinced, finally, that the indicated amount was owed. I then explained that the Plan would issue a memorandum bill and the hospital should let us know whether it would send a check or simply ask us to deduct the debt from future payments.

As it turned out, neither method was satisfactory. "We owe the money," Sister Administrator declared, obviously equating delay with dishonor. "We pay." Whereupon she pulled out a roll of bills, counted out the sum, and insisted that I take it with me, agreeing reluctantly to find a cash receipt form and let me sign for it. The Sisters in this case had arrived in this country only recently as representatives of an Eastern European order, and their methods may have been simpler than most, but it is possible still to cherish the "we owe, we pay" ethic and wish it had enjoyed a longer life.

*Ratio of charges to charges according to cost.

At any rate, it is not to be thought that billfold or pocketbook accounting was the exclusive practice of religious institutions. When the Plan proposed to sponsor a series of lectures on cost accounting for hospitals, the response of the president of the regional hospital council, a dean among administrators at the time, was: "I can't see why this is necessary. Either you're going along all right, or you aren't going along all right, and that's all there is to it." The president was outvoted, eventually, and the lectures were presented, but all that was less than 40 years ago, and the distance from "we owe, we pay" to RCCAC seems more like from here to eternity.

These 40 years have seen the same kind of quantum jump in every phase of hospital management, operations, and, most dramatically, professional practice. In fact, it may be that the element of the hospital that has changed least over this time is the board of trustees. Different as it is in composition and function, and especially in the scope of its responsibilities, the board today in many ways looks much the same as it did 40 years ago. Trustee work habits have been extended and intensified to accommodate the new worries but have not otherwise undergone radical change. The relationship of the board to management and medical staff has changed, to be sure, but the change is more of degree than of kind. What was changed most of all is the board's accountability, the impact on its deliberations and decisions of things external to the institution: technology, law, bureaucracy, paying and planning agencies, unions, employers, neighbors, communities, the press, and the public.

An examination of the new accountabilities and their effect on how trustees perform was a principal focus of the study reported here, but not the whole of it. In 30 years of reporting hospital and medical affairs I have had many opportunities to observe trustees in their native habitat, and it is the sum of all these observations and impressions, as well as the interviews and conversations and meetings that were undertaken in the preparation of this account of what trustees are up to, that provides the perspective from which this book was written. The approach throughout is journalistic, describing the forces at play in the field and the problems they present, and reporting what trustees themselves, and others inside and outside hospitals whose views are relevant, are thinking and saying and doing about the forces and problems. Thus the method is reportorial, but it should be understood that there is no pretense here that it is therefore objective. In fact, objectivity in reporting is largely a myth anyway; wherever the information comes from, every line the reporter writes passes through a subjective filter and necessarily includes an element of opinion. The goal therefore is not really objectivity, which is impossible to achieve on the face of it, but fairness, which is not impossible but always difficult, because Paul's blessing is Peter's blister. Besides, there are always occasions, here and elsewhere, when a reporter feels constrained to make his own estimate of the truth on the basis of his own observations; where opinion thus obtrudes in these pages, I hope it will be clear that it is mine.

In the course of marshaling my scattered resources for this exercise, I attended a dozen or so hospital board or executive committee meetings, several regional or local conferences of hospital trustees, formal meetings of hospital associations and related groups where organized worrying is the outcome, if not the goal, of the occasion, and the usual number of corridor and hotel room consultations that go with or come after any of these. I also had extended interviews with some 50 trustees, physicians, administrators, and others, including several whose interest would have to be subsumed under the overworked rubric "consumer representative." In all these encounters, and in picking my way through the heavy under-brush of books, articles, monographs, reports, pamphlets, and papers that have been written for or about hospital trustees, in which another twig is hereby entwined to be tugged at by the next explorer, I was seeking, and sometimes finding, elucidation of the interests and problems of the species, the methods and relationships, the satisfactions and anxieties, the triumphs and failures.

Since this was to be an account of how hospital trustees are coping with their problems in the real world, I had intended to name names, places, and dates, as a reporter should and always would like to do, but it became apparent quickly that if this were to be done, what came out would be bleached pale of meaning, devoid of stress and conflict, and thus short of the truth, like a child's garden of verses view of the world. But there are two risks involved in abandoning names, except where people have been willing to talk or write for the record, and resorting elsewhere to such nonattribution as occurs in the anonymous and abbreviated but otherwise true reports of board meetings in chapter 1 and in devices like "one trustee said" and "a physician told a reporter," which I have also used extensively, if reluctantly, here. One risk is that the reader must lean heavily on the reporter's credibility, because there is no other way to determine whether what is reported is what was actually said. The second risk is that in the shelter of anonymity those being interviewed may tend to dwell on conflict and let it all come out, and the resulting report may make it appear that a well-run and essentially harmonious institution is a hotbed of discord.

Like every reporter who has recourse to unnamed sources, I must leave it to the reader to judge the truth for himself, considering not who said it, but what was said. As St. Augustine said of those who disagreed with his interpretation of Moses but didn't deny that both opinions might be right, "I love what they say when they say true, not because it is theirs but because it is true; seeing truth is neither mine, nor his, nor another's, but belonging to us all." This is as good a guide as any, too, for those who may consider that my sources and I have emphasized strife and given harmony short shrift, and thus distorted truth, especially in reporting what is said and done concerning doctor-hospital interests and relationships, and I expect this may be so. Obviously, conversations with a few people over a few months, and at most a few hundred over all the years, in a field of thousands, are not to be considered as representative of anything but themselves. There is no intention to suggest that the problems and conflicts are happening all over, although I believe myself that they are not so rare as some encomiasts for the system have insisted. But I suppose it is possible that this and other reports of hospital events and opinions may indeed exaggerate the incidence of restlessness, not to say mutiny, among the Good Samaritans, because trouble is generally what gets talked about at the meetings and asked about in the interviews and reported in the journals and news columns.

This is not bad, because failure is a lot more instructive than success; nobody really knows why things go smoothly, but everybody learns by examining what went wrong. Nervous trustees and administrators and physicians who protest that airing disputes may hurt the hospital's image and undermine public confidence in hospitals and doctors probably underestimate the public's intelligence. People have better sense than to read a headline about a malpractice suit and conclude that all doctors are incompetent, and even if they did, how are we ever going to solve the problems unless we talk about them? I remember a Clinical Congress of the American College of Surgeons, some 20 years ago, when Carl W. Walter, M.D., then a professor of surgery at Harvard who was regarded as one of the world's leading authorities on operating room asepsis, presented a lecture excoriating the surgeons for laxity in the enforcement of aseptic technique in their hospitals. He showed examples, on slides, of unthinkable lapses in the most respectable institutions, and the surgeons nodded their heads and agreed that things were pretty bad. "Carl is right, you know, we've got to tighten up," they told one another soberly as they left the lecture hall.

Then, in keeping with the college's policy of conducting open meetings, Dr. Walter repeated his charges of laxity at a press conference. "Top surgeon says hospitals are pigsties," said the headline in the afternoon newspaper, and within hours the wire services were carrying the story all over the country. That was exactly what he had said, and the surgeons were furious. "Outrageous, irresponsible, unethical" were among the nicer things they said about Dr. Walter, and letters that came to the college predicted that people would be afraid to go to hospitals, fail to get needed surgery, and die. They stopped short of accusing Dr. Walter of murder, but just barely.

Well, people are not that dumb. Carl Walter was never addicted to understatement, to be sure, and he might readily have found some less abrasive way of making his point, but it is unlikely that a single person among the millions who read the headlines could have considered that operating rooms looked like pigsties, or anything else except the truth—that a leading authority on the subject was disturbed enough about conditions to choose this method of prodding his colleagues to take action. Moreover, if Dr. Walter had stated the case conservatively, it wouldn't have attracted any notice at all, and the surgeons and administrators and operating room supervisors who were shocked by the newspaper stories into investigating practices at their own hospitals wouldn't have done anything, and conditions might have got worse instead of better. Of course, there isn't any possible way to measure either the good or bad effects of this kind of episode and thus strike a balance between the damage and the improvement that may result. You believe what you want to believe. I believe that the Carl Walter strictures, and the few critical observations included in this report, are good for hospitals, on balance. A lot of people disagreed with me then, and I expect some will now.

At any rate, it should be clear by this time that the purpose of this book is neither to pat heads nor to solve problems. It is not a panegyric celebrating the wisdom and nobility of all those whose labors aid the sick and injured, nor an encyclopedia of the accumulated knowledge about hospitals and trustees, nor yet a textbook trustees can use, like the Yellow Pages, to look up answers to their problems. There are panegyrics and encyclopedias and textbooks enough to satisfy the needs of any seekers after praise or knowledge or answers. But it has been my impression that most of these gather dust on library shelves, and so there might be a need for something trustees would read—and possibly even enjoy reading—that would provide glimpses, at least, of how others are confronting the forces and coping with the problems all hospitals face. There are few prescriptions, or "should do's," here, except as I have reported what those with some professional or administrative or official authority have said should be done, and I am inclined to be suspicious even of these, because the rise to authority is often achieved, as Bertrand Russell once said, "by those who feel the strongest certainty about matters on which doubt is the only rational attitude." The same suspicion, for the same reason, should apply in the case of the few "should do's" of my own, which appear in the chapter on public relations, a field in which I have practiced enough to understand that doubt is the only rational attitude toward almost any proposition that may be advanced.

Several years ago, I wrote a book that was concerned, as this one is, with doctors and hospitals, and Medicare and Medicaid, and Blue Cross, and planning, and all the other arcana that must be some part of the life and interest of anybody who is likely to be reading these pages. In due course the book was reviewed, as such books are, in the *Journal of the American Medical Association*. The physician who wrote the review was a man who didn't know me, and I didn't know him, but he said in his review that he thought I was a competent observer of medical affairs and what I had to say was for the most part accurate and fair. At about the same time, the same book was reviewed in *Medical World News,* and in this case the review was written by the editor, Morris Fishbein, M.D. I have known Dr. Fishbein for more than 30 years, and he has known me for more than 30 years, and he said in his review that I was "uninformed and impertinent."

Now I am not qualified to say which of these two divergent views may be closer to the truth, though I must say I have a definite preference, but I do suggest that the reader would be well advised to keep them both in mind as he prepares now to moisten a finger and raise it to see which way the wind is blowing. That finger already up there is mine.

1.

WILL THE MEETING PLEASE COME TO ORDER?

YOU HAVE TO HAVE THE BACKUP

Upstairs in the patients' rooms tonight there are 344 souls, nearly all in some kind of trouble or discomfort. A few are critically ill, hurting and frightened, taking solace as they can from the men and women who are there to help. Twenty-two were operated on today. Four of them got up well this morning at home and went about their business until mischance struck them down and brought them to the emergency department, where 112 others were also treated today. Five of them are there now; they were in an accident on the tollway earlier this evening; soon the night staff in radiology will report whether two of them can be released or must be admitted to the hospital for further examination and treatment tomorrow.

Outside the emergency rooms, down the corridor just a few steps, the brightly lit, cheerfully furnished lobby is busy with visitors coming and going, some just waiting. Many stop at the information counter across from the entrance, where women in pink and white uniforms listen patiently to questions, find answers, offer suggestions. These are volunteers. Twenty of them are on duty here and elsewhere in the hospital tonight. They have chosen to be at the hospital working. They are not paid, except as they may consider it in some way rewarding to be, and feel, useful.

The same thing is true of the men here in the boardroom, where they have come for a meeting of the executive committee of the hospital's board of directors. Like the corridor and lobby, the boardroom is light and cheery, paneled in a light wood, with a huge round table of the same finish. The chairs are upholstered and comfortable, but not lavish. The effect is not Wall Street, but it is not Main Street, either—somewhere in between, like the suburban community the hospital serves. Like the community, too, the hospital is growing: a 150-bed addition is almost completed, and the committee tonight will receive an auditor's report of the financing plans for further construction and modernization. The east lawn and part of the parking lot have given way to the contractor's trailer offices and equipment shacks while the addition was under construction, and they will be here again for the next step. It has been almost a constant condition of life for this institution, now in its 25th year.

The meeting is scheduled for 7:30, and the members are drifting in one at a time with a few minutes to spare, taking places at the near side of the round table. There will be just 10 members here tonight, all men, and there is some joking about the four or five absentees, presumably taking their ease in the sun while the faithful toil. The group here now is mostly middle-aged. Only two members are noticeably gray. The chairman of the board might be called early elderly, as somebody has delicately described it, and one member, the hospital administrator, is visibly younger than the others. Actually, he is 35. Just two of these men wear the dark suit that is the uniform of boardrooms downtown. Light gray and tan weaves are preferred here, and there are several in sports coats, including the administrator.

At exactly 7:30 the two physician members come in and sit together, and the chairman calls the meeting to order. The minutes of the last meeting are approved.

The first business is the report of the finance committee, which includes the report of an auditor's review of the financing for the new construction. The report is for information only; it has been circulated to the members in advance of this meeting, and there are no questions. The only comment is the chairman's. "It's a good report," he says, "a clear explanation of the program we were so concerned with during the summer and fall. It looks just as we thought it would." The basic instrument described in the auditor's report is a new $20 million hospital facility revenue bond issue that was used to retire the outstanding bonds and set up an interim construction fund for completion of the addition and several planned modernization projects, including a new intensive care unit. With the issuance of the new bonds, the hospital conveyed its buildings and land to the city and is leasing them back until the bonds are retired, when the property will revert to hospital ownership. That will be October 1, 2001. For the first two months of this year, the finance committee chairman reports, operating expenses were below budget. Everybody looks pleased, and there are murmurs of approval.

A foundation committee has had a meeting to assign fund-raising responsibilities among its members, two of whom are present. One has called on all the names assigned to him and says vaguely that "the response is all we hoped for." The other member hasn't called on his names yet. No questions, no comments. In its reasonably affluent community, this hospital does well with its fund raising, but it is the stuff of the auditor's report, not the fund-raising committee, that fuels the hospital's capital expansion today.

The physicians on the executive committee are the president and the vice-president of the medical staff, and the president-elect of the staff is a member of the board of directors, but not of this committee. "They're members as officers of the staff, representing the staff," the hospital administrator has explained to a friend. "To pretend that staff physicians can be directors and *not* represent the staff, as some consultants and authorities have recommended, is playing games. It just doesn't work out that way."

When the medical report is called for, the vice-president of the staff begins by going directly to a touchy matter of credentials: an application for privileges that the staff has recommended should be rejected. The stated reasons are that the applicant's credentials, which are described as "average," are not up to the standards of the department to which he has applied. Besides, the doctor making the report adds, "His office is in another suburb several miles away, and this would not be his primary hospital."

The administrator's title is president. He is a voting member of the board of directors and the executive committee, and he opposes the staff recommendation. "Those reasons aren't good enough," he says. " 'Average credentials' and 'not up to our standards' have got to be stated in specific terms. The applicant is board eligible. What *are* our standards? Considerations of personality have to be ruled out unless there are questions about qualifications. Also, the fact that his office isn't nearby can't be considered relevant. The question is, can he serve our patients here? I've asked for legal advice on these questions, and I think we should hold up any action on this application until the lawyers' opinion is presented to the joint conference committee at its meeting next month. First, all the legal requirements have to be examined, and then we have to develop a policy, with written standards. These don't necessarily have to be the same for all departments of the staff, but they have to be specific in every case. I move we defer action on the application until we have the legal opinion and the staff as a whole has had an opportunity to consider it." The motion is seconded.

The doctors are silent, but another committee member protests that postponement won't accomplish anything. "It will take months to go through all that," he suggests, "and then we'll be back here considering the same question we have now. Do we want this man, or not?"

The president persists. "The staff says it doesn't want him," he points out, "but we can't brush him off by saying that his qualifications aren't up to our standards. What do we mean by that? We have to have better reasons than the ones that have been stated here. We need clear understanding, by the entire medical staff, of our legal responsibilities in dealing with credentials."

The board member who has objected to postponement is a line executive of a large corporation. He has heard all this before, and he is persistent, too. "We don't have to do everything the lawyers tell us we should," he objects. "We'd never get anything done."

The president of the medical staff, a surgeon, makes a joke. "You're not as afraid of lawyers as we have to be," he says to the board member.

The president of the hospital isn't joking. "We turned down an applicant for another department a year ago," he reminds the committee, "and there's no way we could substantiate that action now if the man should come back at us. We mustn't do that again, even if it should take us two or three months to find out everything we need to know." He adds another hint of what lies beneath the surface of this discussion: "We can't turn a man down simply because we think we might have trouble with him."

Now the surgeon isn't joking either. "I have a gut feeling about this," he says, "and our gut feelings have usually been right. You can nearly always pick out the ones who are going to cause trouble."

The discussion isn't going anywhere, and the chairman calls for a vote on the president's motion to postpone action until the lawyers' report can be presented to the joint conference committee. Nobody votes no.

Next, the president reports that the Joint Commission on Accreditation of Hospitals has scheduled a survey of the hospital. It will take two days, and the key issues being looked at are peer review and medical audits. At JCAH and elsewhere in medical circles, quality assurance is the height of fashion this year. "We're in pretty good shape," the president tells the committee. "Our review and audit procedures have been improving right along in all departments. I don't see that we can have any problems with the Joint Commission."

The chairman repeats the dates of the survey and urges members of the board to attend, at least for the opening meeting on the first day of the survey, when the JCAH surveyors meet with representatives of the staff and administration to outline the procedure that will be followed. "The surveyors are favorably impressed when board members attend these meetings," the chairman says. "You'll get a feeling for what they're interested in and what they're looking for. It's important for as many of you as can possibly make it to be there for that meeting, at least." Somebody wants to know what time the meeting will start. The chairman recalls that it has usually been around 9:30, and there is some kidding about bankers' hours. The president adds that it's equally important for directors to attend the review session at the end of the second day, when the surveyors comment on their impressions and answer questions from the staff.

Continuing with his report as chief operating executive, the president mentions the problem of malpractice insurance, which has everybody rattled right now. The hospital contracts with a medical group for emergency service, and members of the group are having difficulty getting adequate insurance coverage. The hospital and the contractors have been named as joint defendants in some suits, and thus the matter of their coverage is important. "We need to be just as particular about the qualifications of the emergency department physicians as we are about our own staff," the president warns. A nearby hospital has had to include its emergency department physicians in its own coverage because they couldn't get satisfactory malpractice insurance themselves. "The same thing could happen to us," he concludes. "There are sure to be further serious questions about hospital and physician malpractice insurance. It's a national problem. The amount of our own premiums seems high to us, but as a percentage of the hospital budget it's much smaller than the percentage of their incomes doctors are having to pay for malpractice insurance today."

Now the president turns to a matter of medical quality: the stiffened requirements for utilization review of Medicare patients. It has been proposed that review to certify necessity of care should be conducted within one working day following admission, and there are new requirements for written criteria and standards, recertification of continued stays, and medical care evaluation. It's going to take a lot of time, and the staff wants the hospital to hire physicians to get it done. But the president thinks utilization review should be kept within the hospital's own medical staff. "Contracting this function to outside physicians would invite interference," he argues. The whole matter has been discussed at a meeting of the medical staff, where he and the staff president took opposing positions, and the issue was debated at length. The staff finally voted to continue doing its own utilization review, as it had been doing before the new requirements were announced. "But it was a close vote," the president says, looking across the table at the surgeon, who hasn't commented. Everybody understands that this is going to come up again.

There are also some problems with the hospital's arrangement for anesthesiology services, the president tells the committee. Two groups of anesthesiologists are under contract, and there have been some difficulties about space and scheduling. "We hope to get them working together more effectively," he adds. Nobody is inclined to ask for any more details, and he goes on to mention that a new medical director for respiratory therapy is proving to be competent and energetic and is working on plans for a pulmonary function laboratory. Everybody is happy with the way this department is going, and there are hopes that the job can be expanded so there will be one medical director for all intensive care services.

As it turns out, however, nobody is especially happy with the state of affairs in another department. The staff has expressed displeasure with the quality of the services. Consultants have been called in to examine the entire program and make recommendations for change, and there will be another report when their studies are completed. The doctors don't have anything to say about this, but they spring to eager attention, like bird dogs on a point, when the president reports that a team from the hospital has visited a hospital in another city to study the cardiac surgery and angiography facilities and services. "The price is high," he cautions, "and more investigation is needed. Also, the new planning law gives the state planning agency the authority to make certain that 'only those services, facilities, and organizations found to be needed shall be offered or developed in the state.' They're zeroing in on services, and they're certain to be looking at cardiac surgery."

Now the surgeon leans forward. "We have to keep up," he declares. "Our emergency department is a great resource. We can do anything. The other day we had a young girl—a bad accident—with a torn aorta. Her life was saved. But we have to have the facilities. If you're going to be out in front, you have to have the backup!" He pauses, then leans back and adds thoughtfully, "You know, we didn't start out here to become a hospital that would do everything, but we may be forced into it. The only cases we're transferring to other hospitals now are severe burns and some neurosurgery."

Heads nod around the table, and the president reminds the committee that the hospital's emergency services have made it a designated trauma center, the highest classification in the state's emergency service network. The hospital has pioneered in initiating a regional system for handling cardiac emergencies, with communication to the hospital by telemetry from specially equipped ambulances. A public opinion survey has indicated rising awareness of the value of these emergency services to the community. "The survey response also shows that waiting time in the emergency department has been reduced," the president adds.

No action is called for, but the discussion has reminded him of a troublesome detail. "As you know, we have all the needed planning approvals for our intensive care addition," he says. "The regional, state, and federal planning authorities have looked at what we intend to do and said go ahead. But now, under a new ordinance it seems we also have to have the approval of the village planning board." Somebody wants to know whether there is a fee involved in obtaining the local review and approval, and the president says no. "It's just another hoop we have to jump through," he comments.

He has one more announcement. "We're interviewing applicants for a staff chaplaincy," he reports. The surgeon asks if it will be a full-time job, and the answer is yes. "Some hospitals our size have two or three chaplains," the president explains. "So," remarks the surgeon, "he'll have a flock but not a church. I suppose now we'll have to enlarge the two-seat chapel." It is a reference to the customary retiring room for anxious and bereaved families. The remark is good natured, and there has been no tension here, but a message has been sent and received: the staff considers some hospital services more important than others.

The chairman reports now that the directors of the hospital's pension fund as fiduciary trustees and the president as fiduciary agent for the finance committee have to be bonded. There is no further comment, no more old business, no new business, and the meeting is adjourned. It is 8:50 p.m.

THE STUDY IS GOING FORWARD

This is the executive committee of a big city medical center—a formidable cross section of the city's business and financial power structure. In fact, there are only two other boards in the city—one hospital, one university—whose concentration of wealth, power, and social position might exceed this one's. Secure at the pinnacle of power, the other boards, like some corporations, have reached out to season their WASP flavor with a dash of alien culture. The money on this board isn't quite that old. You can usually tell old money by looking down the roster and seeing how many of the given names are also obviously family names. Thus Allen McAlester might be anybody, but McAlester Allen, or McAlester Allen III, is probably *somebody*. The method isn't infallible, but it is usually indicative.

The committee is meeting for luncheon at a downtown club—a circumstance that pains one or two older board members who like the hospital atmosphere and think something is lost when board members meet elsewhere. The board itself, which has an abundant 50 members, meets quarterly in the hospital auditorium. These are formal, ceremonial occasions. The business of the institution is conducted by the 20-member executive committee, and experience has shown that attendance is notably better when the meetings are held here; these are people who count minutes.

There are 16 members today. Each one finds beside his place a maroon binder with a copy of the day's agenda and the appropriate backup materials, including current operating statistics and a list of the month's gifts, grants, and bequests. These total $104,206—an average month. As the committee members come in and take their places they greet one another briefly, then pick up their folders and glance at the reports.

"When you don't admit so many you keep 'em longer, is that it?" says one, looking across the table at the hospital's chief executive and grinning. The president grins back. "That's the idea," he says. They both know the variations here are so slight as to be meaningless, but they enjoy the fact that the board member has been quick to spot a key statistical datum: admissions are down, and length of stay is up.

There are two physicians present. One is dean of the medical school the hospital is affiliated with, and the other is a surgical specialist on the hospital staff and medical school faculty, who enlivens the occasion with a report of a conversation he has had with a young friend of his son's, a consumer activist whose group is planning to investigate hospitals. "He wanted to know who gets all the loot," the surgeon says. "I tried to tell him that isn't the way it works, but I didn't get anywhere. He was absolutely convinced that somebody is 'ripping off millions,' and he wasn't going to believe anything to the contrary." Some of the young medical students and house staff members have much the same idea, the surgeon adds.

The reaction to all this is generally more amused or resigned than dismayed, but one board member is outraged. Interestingly, he is one of the younger members of this middle-aged group. "What can we do to combat this kind of ignorance?" he wants to know. "Can't we even teach the fundamentals of hospital economics to our own medical students?"

The dean has been here before. "It's been tried," he says. "But it has to be offered as an elective, given the demands on the curriculum, and the students just aren't that interested. The subject is too far removed from their needs and concerns of the moment."

The board member doesn't give up. "But they do have to learn something about the business of running a medical practice, don't they?" he asks. "Couldn't the hospital side be presented along with that?"

The economics of private practice are even more remote from the interests of medical students than hospital business is, the dean explains, and the surgeon adds that this remains true throughout the internship and residency years, and even beyond, inasmuch as increasing numbers of young physicians go on from their residencies into fellowships, group practices, or associations with physicians whose practices are already established. The number who enter private practice by themselves has been shrinking for a generation. The young physicians always have their eyes on the next step: a residency, fellowship, board exams, another appointment. The business side of practice is something for somebody else to worry about.

The young board member is still troubled about this, but he doesn't pursue the matter any further as the business of the meeting gets under way with the ritual motion to approve the minutes of the last meeting and the ritual response. A recommended change in rank for a member of the medical staff is approved in the time it takes to read it, and the committee's attention is turned to a proposal for the medical center of which the hospital is a part to undertake a feasibility study looking toward possible establishment of a health maintenance organization.

The plan calls for the medical center to hire a consultant, and the proposal includes an agreement that the medical center institutions will take actions relating to HMOs only with full information and approval of the medical center board. This part of the proposal, the president of the hospital points out, marks the first time the medical center corporation has asked its member institutions for any such binding agreement.

"This is the time to find out whether you've got a medical center that wants to go out and do something, or just a social club," the president says. The hospital's share of the HMO planning budget is estimated to be $30,000. There are no questions, and authorization of the hospital's participation in the proposed study is approved, on motion by the young board member who is worried about medical students.

Another set of medical center proposals has to do with teaching and consulting affiliations with nonmember institutions and transfers of patients to the medical center. Again, the proposals seek coordinated planning and ask for agreement on all institutional affiliations. The president explains that other medical schools with downtown hospitals have been pursuing clinical teaching affiliations with community hospitals in suburbs and outlying areas, and one or two of these affiliations appear to encroach on the suburban area from which referrals to this hospital have traditionally been made.

"These resolutions say, 'Let's get about the business of investigating affiliations and do it through the medical center,' " he concludes, triggering a lively discussion of the areas and institutions involved. It is obvious that a competitive nerve has been touched. Everybody is alert to the implications as the president reviews the referral channels that have already been occupied or explored by the other groups.

"What's left?" somebody wants to know, and it turns out that while the number of suburban hospitals is not unlimited, there is still a lot of unplowed territory out there.

"What have we got to offer?" a board member asks. Students, house staff, faculty consultants.

What can they offer us? Referrals, mostly. Also, it's another dimension to the learning experience of medical students and house staff. The community hospital is part of the real world of medical practice.

Could we act fast if we decided to move? Yes.

Nobody asks what expense may be involved. The fact that referrals may be at risk is enough for this group of bankers, businessmen, and lawyers.

The dean explains that patterns of physician behavior are involved. "Some of these people may be leaning toward us, some toward the other medical schools. Some don't want to be bothered." The president mentions that the National Health Planning and Resources Development Act will shift the planning emphasis from bed control to service systems. There will be a plan for the area, and tertiary care centers will be designated. "There may be some unhappy institutions," he concludes.

Motion to approve the proposals. Passed. It won't be us.

The chairman calls for the report of the finance committee, which has been authorized to select a firm to make a feasibility study for financing the hospital's long-term capital expansion. The amount is $40 million. The committee has interviewed representatives of several firms, the chairman reports, and was especially impressed with the presentation made by a well-known management consultant. However, another firm was selected, finally, because of its superior qualifications and experience with this type of hospital finance. In fact, this firm has recently done a study for another medical center in the city. Nods and smiles as the competitive nerve is nudged again. The study is going forward.

Meanwhile, the hospital needs $8 million this year to complete some structural alterations and modernization within the present plant, the finance chairman explains. The committee is considering two alternatives. One is a loan from a downtown bank, at the prime rate plus a half, to be replaced by a proposed issue of state health authority tax-exempt bonds, which the bank would then undertake to sell. The other alternative is a short-term health authority note that could be converted to the tax-exempt bonds. The authority note appears to be more economical, but without getting the loan the downtown bank would take only a fraction of the bonds, so the first method might be more desirable. Pending completion of the feasibility study, the finance chairman wants to talk to a couple of other banks. He's been looking over their statements and has a feeling they might be interested in the tax-exempt bonds.

The only question has to do with repayment of the short-term loan, which can be refinanced until the long-term credit is arranged. Forty million is the outside figure; it may be cut back by the ongoing fund-raising effort. Nobody doubts that the building program will go forward on schedule. The interest charges alone will come to $10 a patient-day.

Now the chairman reports for a search committee that is sifting candidates to succeed the hospital president, who will retire in a few years. The committee has engaged an executive search consultant who has been on the job for a month and has screened the list down to about 30 candidates. In another six weeks or so the consultant expects to recommend a few candidates for interviews with the committee. The list still includes some with mostly business experience, some physicians, and some trained and experienced as hospital executives.

Next on the agenda is the report of the president. He has been visited by a delegation of house staff representatives seeking recognition as a collective bargaining unit, now permitted under recent amendments to the National Labor Relations Act. The medical center has a Joint House Staff Council, but the decision to recognize is up to the institution. Are interns and residents employees, or are they students? A Pennsylvania court has said students, but a Michigan court has just ruled the other way. This issue is now before the National Labor Relations Board, and a ruling is expected shortly.

Meanwhile, the joint council has asked for a raise in interns' salaries from $11,700 to $16,500, beginning with the new intern class in July. The hospitals have offered $12,200. "It is one thing to negotiate salaries," says the president, who will do the negotiating and make the decision without seeking instruction from the committee, "but recognition is something else. When that happens, you have an organization that wants to talk about patient services, representation on staff committees. Some places, they've demanded membership on the board. You'd be interested to sit in on some of our meetings with these young people."

Not really. The recognition issue will come to the committee again. "They are not naive," the dean warns, "and they have excellent counsel."

The meeting ends with a report from the chairman of the fund-raising committee, who calls attention to the gifts and bequests listed in the monthly report. The amount is impressive, but it isn't $40 million. Adjourned.

WE MAY GET SOME, BUT
WE WON'T GET IT ALL

The hospital board of directors has 28 members, and 22 of them are here today for the regular monthly meeting, along with half a dozen members of the hospital's administrative staff. They are sitting around the outside of a hollow rectangle made of narrow tables set up in an all-purpose meeting room on the top floor of one of the hospital's older buildings. A film projector, overhead projector, TV set, viewing screen, and blackboard have been pushed out of the way at one end of the room; these are used at meetings of the medical and nursing staffs, but they are not needed today. The room is crowded, and a latecomer has perched on a table in a corner, but the impression is not so much of untidiness as of a no-nonsense workroom. The floor is black and white composition tile, well worn.

The hospital is one of three serving a city of 200,000 population whose largest industry is state government. The city also has its share of diversified manufacture, and the leading companies are represented here, along with community leaders in banking, insurance, and law. Two members of the board are physicians, and three are women. The city has a sizable black population, and there are two black directors here. The hospital administrator is also a member of the board, whose president is a retired utilities executive. This is a thin, quiet-spoken gentleman whose manner reminds one of what used to be called "a touch of old-world courtesy." The term, like the manner, is not abundantly evident in today's society.

The president—a board member who has not relinquished the title to the administrator, as many have done—opens the meeting by asking those present to bow their heads while he delivers a brief, modest petition seeking divine guidance for this group as it gets on with its mission of aiding the sick and injured. This is not a church-related institution, but, like most others, it needs all the help it can get.

Three newly elected board members are attending their first meeting today, and the president introduces them formally, remarking on the obvious fact that two of them are considerably younger than most of the directors. There is some joking about this with the third new member, who protests that he is not yet ready to be written off to Medicare. Here as elsewhere, however, there is a discernible effort to replace older members of hospital boards as they retire with young people whose lifetime of service is still ahead of them and who, it is believed, though it isn't always true, are readier to accommodate the changes and demands a restless society is pressing on its institutions.

The real business of the meeting begins with the report of the treasurer, who asks the members to refer to the balance sheet that is the first page in a bulky loose-leaf notebook that has been given to each of the directors. He calls attention to the fact that cash on hand has been reduced by an amount used for land acquisition. The hospital has been buying up property on an adjacent street; one or two parcels remain to clear the way for the next step in the building program, which is already well advanced in planning.

The next page in the notebook is an analysis of accounts receivable, and the treasurer points out that receivables total approximately $500,000 more than the total at the end of the corresponding month last year, a circumstance reflecting changes in the economy: Medicare and Medicaid payments are slower than they were a year ago, for one thing, and in fact all classes of payment show some increase in receivables. The treasurer reads the figures line by line and then summarizes the analysis showing aggregate receivables at 52 days of outstanding income, compared to 42 days at this time last year. "It is important for us to correct this 25 percent increase," he comments. "It won't be easy to do. We may have to add a person to the collection staff, or reorganize the work. The amount has to be reduced."

He turns the page now to the statement of income and expense, and most of the directors turn the page with him and follow his remarks down the column for the current month, noting the comparisons with last month and last year. Operating income is a little ahead of last year, and a little ahead of budget. Expenses are up, too, but not as much as had been expected. The net gain from operations is healthy, and the loss after depreciation has been charged is minuscule.

Before the board can relax, however, the treasurer adds a note of caution. State law now gives the commissioner of public health the authority to approve rates paid to hospitals by Medicaid and Blue Cross, he reminds the members, and the commission has just notified the hospital this week that its request for approval of the rate for the current year has been reduced by $8 per patient per day.

"We expect to file an answer supporting our request," the treasurer adds. "We may get some of the difference back, but we won't get it all." At the rate the commissioner has established, the hospital would lose $400,000 a year on its Medicaid and Blue Cross payments. "We can't live with that," he declares. "We'll have to get our expenses in line with the actual rate."

Now the president reports that he and another board member have spent most of the day at a meeting of the regional hospital council. "There were 11 items on the agenda," he says, "but we spent three-quarters of the meeting discussing this rate problem. All the hospitals have been cut back—some more than we were, some less. In one case the cutback was $25 a day. Nobody knows what to do, but first we have to go through all the steps: protest, present all the facts, wait for an answer, then appeal if we must."

He turns to the three new directors who are sitting together at his right. "The hospital isn't going broke," he says gently. "We don't want our new members to worry. But we have to take in what we pay out. We can't operate at a loss."

In reply to a question about the appeal procedure, one of the lawyers explains that *last year's* rate at several hospitals has never been satisfactorily adjudicated by the commissioner's office. The hospitals have now sued for relief, and the case is about to go to court. The lawyer agrees with the treasurer's judgment. "We may get something back on appeal," he says. "We're better off than most of the hospitals." The president reports that some hospitals have had to put off paying suppliers in order to meet their payrolls, and the lawyer adds that in the case of last year's rates the commissioner's office failed to comply with requirements of the Administrative Procedure Act. Another board member wants to know whether it wouldn't be prudent to anticipate an unfavorable ruling by the commissioner and start right away to cut expenses wherever possible. The treasurer agrees.

But the president resists. "We want to look at all the figures first," he says. "We've just received notice of the tentative rate, and we mustn't act hastily in a way that might curtail services."

Several members speak up for prudence, and there is agreement, finally, that while the appeal is being prepared studies should be undertaken looking toward the need to reduce expense. Now a board member asks why it wouldn't be possible simply to raise rates and thus add to revenues, instead of cutting expense, and at the president's request the administrator explains that 80 percent of the hospital's business is fixed at the state-approved rate or the Medicare rate, which is comparable, and is actually unrelated to the hospital's published charges.

The questioner doesn't subside. "Why don't we raise rates for the other 20 percent," he asks, "and at least get what we can?"

It wouldn't be practical, the administrator explains. The 20 percent includes some charitable cases that don't come under any of the welfare programs and can't pay their own way, and the private patients who do pay are already paying more than their share. But there will be some added revenue from the outpatient department, where volume is increasing, he adds soothingly.

Next is the report of the medical director, who goes quickly through a comparative report of professional performance that is in the directors' notebooks. It shows increased activity in nearly all departments. Admissions and occupancy are up over last month and this month last year; length of stay is down a half day. There are no questions, and the medical director moves to the next page, a report of incomplete and delinquent medical records. The report shows some improvement in the number of delinquent records over the last year, the medical director explains, but there are still too many, and the outside pressures on hospitals for utilization review and quality assessment are such that performance must be improved more. "The guts of all activity in quality assurance is documentation, or good medical records, so we have been enforcing the penalties for delinquency in recent weeks and have actually suspended admissions for several staff members who were seriously in arrears," the director reports.

A board member asks if that resulted in better performance, and the medical director responds delicately that "we're using friendly persuasion."

"Does that answer your question?" the president asks.

"I think so," the board member responds doubtfully.

Before the conversation can be pursued, another member intervenes with another question. He has been studying the performance statistics and has spotted something: the postoperative infection rate for clean cases is reported at 0.661 percent, compared to 0.476 last month. He wonders if there is an explanation. The medical director explains that the rate in both cases is minimal, and it isn't possible to interpret the change without an analysis of individual case reports. "It's not clear what this means," he finishes, and it is understood that another time the analysis of individual case records will precede, not follow, the board meeting.

The medical director concludes his report with a description of continuing medical education programs that have been developed at the hospital. Presentations on TB, hepatitis, diabetes, gynecology, and medical audit procedure have been completed, and others are in preparation. The courses have been planned to make it convenient for staff members to meet the continuing education requirements of their medical and specialty societies with minimum inconvenience and loss of time from their practices, he adds. In reply to a question, he explains briefly what these requirements are: in most cases a minimum number of hours a year of approved postgraduate training.

The administrator reports two bequests to the hospital totaling something more than $100,000 and a gift of $295 for a special mattress that aids treatment of decubitus ulcers. This interests the board members, and they take a few minutes to find out how it works. There are no questions or comments on the bequests.

Now the administrator asks his associate to report the impact on hospital operations of a health maintenance organization that has been initiated by 40 members of the hospital's medical staff, with encouragement and assistance from the administration and the board. The HMO has enrolled 4,000 members in less than a year and expects to add 10,000 in the next year, the associate explains. He gives figures for the number of inpatient days and various outpatient services the hospital has rendered for members of the group and suggests that the HMO has obviously contributed to the increases in hospital volume. "But we can't be sure, of course, that these people wouldn't have come to us for these services anyway," he adds. Comparing the HMO group's use of services with utilization figures furnished by Blue Cross shows the HMO members use significantly fewer hospital days per 1,000 of covered population, he explains.

"But you can't tell how many of these people would have gone elsewhere if they hadn't joined our HMO?" the president asks.

"No," replies the associate administrator. The president smiles. "Forgive me for asking such a competitive question," he says.

Now the questions fly. How is the hospital being paid? Flat rate per month per enrollee. How are we coming out? Seems about right. Too early to tell, but the group is growing ahead of expectations. Others being crowded out? No sign of it. Do our expansion plans allow for group utilization? Yes. What about the outpatient services? About as anticipated, adjusted for the growth rate. Is the hospital at risk? Yes, but the rate can be adjused if need be. What about the doctors? Same deal. What about staffing for the increased volume of outpatient services? Good question. It may be necessary to add a primary care physician; new members of the HMO group require a lot of basic tests. Was this considered in the rate? Yes, but maybe not enough. We'll have to see.

The next business on the agenda is the report of the president, who begins by congratulating a member of the board who has been named recipient of the state hospital association's annual achievement award. The recognition is richly deserved, the president adds. "He has served on any number of association committees and boards and has spoken at conferences and represented the association in national affairs," the president explains. The board member acknowledges this with a brief response stressing the importance of group action by hospitals, needed especially now that public authorities are moving into hospital operations, as in the case of the state rate ruling. "We've got to work these problems out together," he declares. Nods of agreement circle the room, but nobody volunteers.

The president reminds the board that the annual nurses' graduation dinner will be held at the hospital next month. He mentions the date and urges everybody who possibly can to attend. "It's been traditional for all the members of the board to come to this dinner," he says, smiling at the new members, "and they always have come." Somebody asks him to repeat the date, and there is a show of pens and datebooks, suggesting that the board has got the message.

Now come the reports of committees. The president leads off by calling attention to the executive committee report, which is in the directors' notebooks. The report mentions the property that has been purchased, but not the amount paid, and a board member wants to know what it was. Eighty-three thousand. No other questions.

The chairman of the nursing committee reports that next year's entering nursing school class is already full, which is extraordinary this early in the year. As is customary, the school has accepted a few more candidates than it wants, to allow for the inevitable dropouts, but the number is small. In contrast to the common experience elsewhere, the school enjoys a high rate of acceptance among candidates selected and a low rate of shrinkage from acceptance to matriculation. There is no need here to play admissions roulette and risk ending with empty seats in the classroom, or more bodies than room.

"You remember that we raised the tuition charge, and some of you thought we might lose some students because of it," the chairman says, "but this experience suggests that we shouldn't hesitate to increase the fees again if we need to. The tuition doesn't meet the cost of operating the school anyway." He adds that the school has purchased some additional audiovisual equipment and reminds the board of the graduation date. A director asks whether the planned expansion of the hospital includes more space for the school of nursing and whether the number of students in the school is to be increased. The chairman says that no increase in either the space or the enrollment is planned but that the school is studying the possibility of an affiliation with a local college that would permit the enrollment of some students in a degree program in nursing. The president adds that the expansion planned for the hospital will not add to the number of beds but will enlarge outpatient and ancillary departments. "We don't need any more beds at this time," he says, "the area has all the beds it requires."

The chairman of the auxiliary makes a brief report the substance of which is that every member of the board of directors is expected to dispose of a book of tickets for the annual hospital benefit raffle. "You can sell the tickets or give them away, as you wish," she says, handing the books around, "as long as you turn in the money." The president adds that they aren't hard to sell.

Then he calls on another committee to report on state association activities. This report reviews the state's position in the malpractice insurance crisis: when a major carrier stopped writing business in the state, the association sponsored a bill that would have provided temporary relief for uninsured physicians and hospitals, but another company has now offered to take on the risks, so the bill has been withdrawn. The committee chairman explains the problem the companies face, with extended liability for new claims whose origin dates back to episodes that happened 10 or more years ago. The association is proceeding with plans for the formation of a "captive company" to underwrite the hospital malpractice risk, he reports, and a number of legislative proposals are under consideration in the legislature and in the Congress. "I feel confident some program will be developed so that hospitals will be insured," he concludes, "either through the organization of a state arbitration board to settle claims, as is being done in some jurisdictions, or possibly by some kind of no-fault or compensation system." There are no questions, and the president comments dryly, "I hope it will come before our insurance expires next summer."

The chairman of the buildings and methods improvement committee presents, one at a time, requests for half a dozen items of equipment to be purchased, ranging from a fetal monitor for the obstetrics department to some smoke detectors and fire doors that are needed to meet code requirements in one of the older buildings. In each case a representative of the department involved has met with the committee, which is recommending that the purchases be approved. They are—one at a time. The total amount is approximately $40,000.

Considered separately is the committee's report that the state has approved the hospital's application for development of a computerized axial tomography project, which required review under the new certification-of-need law. An ad hoc committee representing the board of directors and the medical staff will now carry the plans to completion and bring the project back to the board for final approval. The president observes that a lot of money—several hundred thousand dollars—is involved, as well as cooperation with the other hospitals, and so he has appointed the subcommittee to make certain all aspects of the project are given the most thorough study. "But we ought to go ahead with it if we can," he concluded. "People needing this service now have to go out of town to get it."

The planning and building committee chairman reports that a zoning variance is going to be required for the expansion program, which includes office space for some of the doctors on the hospital staff. A group of applicants for the space has met with the committee and the architects to go over layouts for the offices. The hospital portion of the plan is about ready to move into the working drawing phase, and the hospital consultant has been meeting with architects and engineers to develop details of the mechanical and electrical systems. Any changes from the basic plan that has been approved by the board will be brought back, the chairman assures the members.

A question that came up during the HMO discussion comes up again: Do the plans provide adequate space for the expanding volume of demand in the outpatient department, especially the increase in laboratory procedures? The expansion has already been figured in the plan, the chairman explains, and, besides, "We're not locked in. The plan is so arranged that further space can be added later on if necessary."

There are no more questions, and a physician board member now reports for the joint conference committee, which met a few days ago and reviewed the results of three retrospective audits that had been conducted by a staff audit committee. The diagnoses selected were cystitis, delivery, and sterilization. The records were all in good order, and there were no deviations from standards. However, some problems were found having to do with permissions for sterilization. These need to be dealt with promptly and have been referred to the appropriate staff committee. There is some nervousness about this; slipups in permission procedure can cause legal complications.

The chairman has several recommendations for staff appointments. There are two promotions from the associate to the attending staff, one in medicine and one in OB-GYN, and one of the senior attending surgeons has asked to be named to the honorary active staff. There is another transfer recommendation: from courtesy to attending staff in neurosurgery. The credentials committee has examined the qualifications in each case and recommends approval, which is moved by the chairman of the joint conference committee. The motion is seconded and approved by the board. No questions were asked before the vote, but now one of the lawyers asks for the floor.

"The approval of staff appointments is the greatest responsibility this board has," he says. "We have to delegate responsibility for determining the appropriateness of credentials, privileges, audits, and other medical judgments to the staff. But our accountability for these decisions is not eliminated. We should be inquiring more about these matters, even when it is hard to ask the right questions. We're all interested in good-quality care. Our inquiries are to ensure the best interest of the hospital as a whole, not simply to satisfy ourselves. I've just voted to approve the appointment of this young man to the attending staff in neurosurgery, but I don't really know anything about his credentials, and I don't think that's right."

There is a moment of silence, and everybody looks at the joint conference chairman, who is obviously astonished. He opens the file folder that is on the table in front of him, then closes it again. "I haven't got his credentials here with me," he says.

Another physician board member comes to the rescue. "You can be assured the credentials committee has studied his qualifications, and his record, carefully. Actually, he's doing a lot of the neurosurgery here already, and he also operates at one of the other hospitals. We think he's very good, and so do they."

Now the joint conference chairman gets back in. "The committee has been tightening the requirements on credentials," he explains. "We expect this to be done by the credentials committee. We review what they have done, but if we went into the same detail it would require special meetings. As it is, the committee reviews the privileges of half the staff every year—which means that every staff member is looked at every other year. The committee has to document everything for a new appointment. We make the applicant account for everything he has done every day for the past 10 years. It's very thorough."

The discussion is over, and so is the meeting, but it seems likely that the chairman of the joint conference committee will not make another recommendation for active appointment without bringing the credentials file along.

2. WHERE WE ARE AND HOW WE GOT HERE

In boardrooms, club rooms, committee rooms, offices, and sometimes in cafeterias and corridors, men and women who are members of hospital governing boards gather in meetings like the ones that have been reported here, examining problems, finding solutions or modifications or palliatives, making plans, worrying—coping. The range of their concerns is staggering: One board is bemused by a $250 mattress while another borrows $40 million without blinking; a state official can put a $400,000 hole in one hospital's budget while another's doctors add $500,000 of expense to stay out in front. The problems are all different, but in one way or another they all relate to management, money, or medicine, and most often to all three, with overlays of complexity arising from the multiplicity of laws and regulations constraining hospital planning and operations today, the vagaries of an economy that is sometimes good and sometimes bad and sometimes worse and always uncertain, and the expectations of a population conditioned by television to the routine delivery of miracles.

The management for which hospital boards of trustees or directors are responsible is by no means simple, even though individual hospitals, with few exceptions, are not large as businesses go. But anybody approaching a hospital problem as a business problem, as most trustees do when they are newly appointed to hospital boards, is likely to stumble quickly into one or another of the land mines armed by the differences between business and hospitals. A department is losing money? Only half utilized? Close it. Get rid of it. But wait a minute. This is a service that is needed and not available elsewhere to the population that looks to us for protection. All right, then raise the charges for other departments to cover the losses. Can't do that, either; the third parties pay only costs of services for their own patients. What to do? Maneuver, negotiate, worry, cope.

The new OR supervisor has resigned? The third one this year? What's the matter up there? The *same doctor*? Why *can't* we straighten him out, or throw him out? He doesn't straighten, and there's no basis for formal action. He'd sue us and win, and, besides, he has lots of patients—and he's *good*. Oh.

What's this talk about sharing the pediatric service with Memorial? Aren't they our competitors? In a way. But we're both going down in peds. A combined department is the only answer. Why can't we build ours up? How? It's the birthrate that shows where peds is going: no babies, no doctors.

For years, these and other differences of *mission* (to render service, not make money) and *structure* (no doctors in private practice influence decisions at General Motors) obscured the many similarities between hospitals and business, almost to the point where good management practices were regarded as irrelevant, if not suspect. A trustee who inquired about the reasons this month's deficit exceeded last month's was committing a gaucherie. It was assumed, and often stated, that we had given that much more in services for the needy. Before World War II, cost accounting was unknown to most hospitals; if the subject came up it was dismissed as unseemly in the conduct of a charitable enterprise. Depreciation was a dirty word. Maids and orderlies were generally overworked and underpaid, but probably not so much as interns and nurses were. Nobody was ever fired for mentioning a union of hospital workers, because nobody ever thought of it. Outside of the operating room and the x-ray department, the most complicated machine on the premises was the elevator. The trustees raised the money, by a refined and effective form of begging, and the doctors spent it. The task of management was to keep the buildings warm and dry, keep complaints about the food away from the trustees, and keep out of the doctors' way.

Actually, of course, it was never all that simple. It only seems that way now, in retrospect, because the new forces of technology and law and public expectation that have been rising steadily for the past generation, added to the indigenous confusions of mission and structure, have made the task of running the hospital monumentally difficult. In fact, it has been described by students of management as the most complex assignment of its kind in the entire society; for all their billions, the managers of General Motors are not accountable at the same time to so many interests having such a divergence of goals.

Before going on to examine the impact of the new forces on management and trustee responsibilities, as will be done in later chapters, it is necessary first to consider how we got where we are, beginning back in the times when the hospital was a charitable and religious asylum for the sick poor, whose safety was its only concern. Whatever the nature of the surrounding community, the hospital took no notice of it; the community, in turn, wanted no part of the hospital and shunned it like the plague whose victims it often sheltered. Give or take a wealthy landowner, merchant, or politician whose beneficent interest in the asylum was considered a safe conduct to God's favor, the only persons who saw the inside were the religious who staffed the hospital and the passive peasants who accepted its ministrations and more often than not never saw the outside again.

The thing that began to change the hospital was the rise of medical knowledge, and the event, more than any other, that opened the gates to the outside world was the discovery of ether anesthetic in the mid-19th century, which declassified surgery from the epic to the merely heroic. Not long afterward, the contributions of Lister and Roentgen threw the doors wide open and speeded conversion of the hospital from a charitable asylum to a workshop for the doctor in private practice. For all its growth in number, size, and function, the hospital for the first 30 years of the 20th century remained the native habitat of the surgeon. It was an operating room with attachments, an extension in space of the incision.

Where the scalpel cuts, the dollar follows, and during the workshop years income from patients supplanted philanthropy as the main source of operating revenue. Benefactions built the buildings, equipped the surgeries, furnished the rooms, and usually at the end of the year made up the deficits created in part by patients who couldn't pay their own bills and in part, for reasons that owed something to the notion that charity and cost accounting couldn't dwell comfortably together under the same roof, by bills rendered below cost, a quaint practice that has long since been laid to rest but rises again from the dead on occasion to haunt institutions negotiating reimbursement contracts. Dependent on patients who paid and donors who disposed, hospitals began to take an interest in their communities, but with the exception of the patients and the donors, the communities weren't especially responsive. The religious mystique had given way to the medical mystique, but the institution was still regarded with awe. The coffee might be criticized, but not the doctor.

Change never rests, however, and during those comparatively simple workshop years two seeds were germinating in the hospital—one scientific and one social—whose flowering in our time has been one of the crowning achievements of our civilization but whose roots have also been growing and spreading, sometimes to the point of threatening the foundations of our institutions.

The scientific seed was the beginning of specialism, initiated by the separation of surgery from the rest of medicine in the early 1900s and continuing steadily through the 1920s and 1930s. Then, fueled by the accelerated advance of medical science in World War II, specialization burst out all over in the postwar years, bringing with it a seemingly unending succession of triumphs over death and disease and disability and making every physician as dependent on the organizational and technological resources of the hospital as the surgeons of the earlier era were on its operating tables. But the roots have been growing along with the branches, and some of our cherished values in medicine have been threatened by the inevitable attenuation of the patient-physician relationship that has accompanied the burgeoning specialization. Most often referred to as "the fragmentation of care," this change in a relationship of trust has become a perplexing problem for physicians and for the governance and management of hospitals, and is seen by many as the basic cause of the rising tide of malpractice lawsuits that has threatened to engulf physicians and hospitals in recent years. For many, the trusted friend has vanished, to be replaced by a parade of strangers, and for some, the lawsuit may be as much a means of expressing grief and resentment at the loss as a means of seeking redress or exacting payment.

The social seed was Blue Cross, which was planted in the soil of economic hardship in the 1930s and now spreads its branches over a large segment of the population. Along with the hospitalization insurance whose origin and growth it stimulated, Blue Cross helped make the hospital a routine instrument, instead of an uncommon recourse, for the physician by removing the financial barrier to admission.

Thus specialization and prepayment combined to penetrate the mystique and bring the hospital and the community together as a part of everyday experience, akin more to the school than to the monastery. Again, however, where there are sheltering branches, there are also creeping roots. As the barriers came down and the hospital became a community enterprise, the practice of admitting patients as much for convenience as for treatment began to grow, at first invisibly. In the 1950s, as hospital costs were rising and Blue Cross subscription rates rose accordingly, the problem of unnecessary hospitalization was publicly aired for the first time,* initiating the first efforts to exercise control through hospital utilization committees, forerunners of today's Professional Standards Review Organizations.

Another result of the growth of prepayment and insurance was a gradual shifting in the community's attitude toward the hospital and the hospital's attitude toward the community. For people who were making periodic payments in anticipation of needing the hospital's services, some of the mystery and awe began to wear away, and in its place came a feeling if not of actual proprietorship, at least of vested interest, and with it, inevitably, a disposition to criticize. Along with the articles on laboratory breakthroughs and miracle cures there began to appear articles suggesting error on Mount Olympus. Fee splitting and unnecessary surgery made the headlines alongside the "new hope for millions of sufferers" that had been the standard in earlier, less complicated times. Gods do not tumble easily, and public criticism of hospitals evoked anger and anguish in board rooms and doctors' lounges. But there was recognition, too, that changing methods of practice and payment were giving new meaning to the pious utterance that "the hospital belongs to the community." For the first time, those who said it and those who heard it began to understand that it might be true.

Over these same years, other forces were at work inching hospitals ever closer to the gray area that separates private and public enterprise. Back in 1932, the report of a national Committee on the Costs of Medical Care, over the protests of most of its physician members, had recommended the reorganization of medical practice, medical insurance supported if necessary by tax funds, and expansion of public health services. Physician members submitted a minority report recommending that "the corporate practice of medicine financed through intermediary agencies" should be vigorously opposed as being economically wasteful, inimical to a sustained quality of medical care, and exploitative of the medical profession. An editorial in the *Journal of the American Medical Association* referred to the majority report as "incitement to revolution," and the ensuing furor may have influenced the Congress to omit any mention of health insurance when it approved the

---

*This was in Pennsylvania, where state insurance commissioner Francis Smith in 1957 conducted public hearings in connection with a Blue Cross request for approval of an increase in subscription rates. He asked a series of physician witnesses whether they ever admitted patients to hospitals just so Blue Cross would pay the bills for diagnostic workups that wouldn't be paid for on an outpatient basis. The witnesses insisted that this couldn't happen unless, in their judgment, the patients had to be in the hospital. Then the commissioner called a final witness, I. S. Ravdin, M.D., who at that time was chairman of the Department of Surgery at the University of Pennsylvania School of Medicine, chairman of the Board of Regents of the American College of Surgeons, and President Eisenhower's personal physician. "Do you ever admit patients to the hospital so that Blue Cross will pay the bill?" commissioner Smith asked. "Of course," said Dr. Ravdin, "doesn't everybody?" In an adjudication issued early in 1958, commissioner Smith approved a part of the requested rate increase and instructed Blue Cross to require its hospitals to organize utilization committees like the one at the Sacred Heart Hospital of Allentown, PA, which had been described during the hearings. With a few exceptions, however, the effort was ineffective and the issue was largely ignored until it was raised again in the conditions for participation in Medicare in 1966.
The official transcript of the hearing may not fully support the language of this version, but this is the way it was widely reported at the time by several witnesses, including Dr. Ravdin himself.

original Social Security Act in 1935.[1] An earlier draft of the bill had proposed study and recommendations concerning health insurance among the functions of the Social Security board created by the act.

But the idea that the health and well-being, as well as the subsistence, of the less fortunate are the responsibility of the whole society and should not be left to the vagaries of charitable disposition or the intention and solvency of local authority has been persistent in the United States, as in other Western nations, and proposals for tax-supported health insurance were back in the Congress in the late 1940s. Again, opposition by the medical profession, the insurance industry, and other conservative forces prevailed, and another decade was to pass before the concept surfaced again, this time in the form of proposed legislation providing medical assistance for the aged population. The issue was debated throughout the last two years of the Eisenhower administration, and a limited form of assistance administered by the states was approved by the Congress in 1961. Then came the surge of Great Society legislation enacted during the Johnson administration: the Civil Rights Act, the Elementary and Secondary Education Act, and, finally, the Social Security Amendments of 1965, including Medicare and Medicaid.

An important predecessor to these entitlements, overlooked and virtually unknown outside the field of medicine and hospitals, was the Hill-Burton Act that had been passed by the Congress in 1946 providing federal grants to stimulate hospital construction, which had been neglected during the depression and war years. Over the next 25 years Hill-Burton assistance played a key role in the vast expansion and modernization of the U.S. hospital plant, bringing improved facilities and services to millions of Americans whose community hospitals were outworn or inadequate and other millions in remote rural areas and spreading suburbs where new hospitals were built.

Although voices other than commissioner Smith's had been raised occasionally over the years to suggest the possibility that more hospitals, more beds, more Blue Cross, and more insurance might result in more use of hospital services than was absolutely necessary, such warnings were generally overlooked or disregarded in the urge to bring better care to more people, and the American disposition to equate "more" and "better" prevailed. Even when, in the mid-1950s, a few studies revealed that a measurable fraction of hospital patients might have been cared for adequately in outpatient departments or doctors' offices, and when the American College of Surgeons issued statements asserting that unnecessary or unjustified surgery was becoming a disciplinary problem within the profession, these findings were generally considered to be aberrations. The Joint Commission on Accreditation of Hospitals had been organized in 1952 by the American Hospital Association, American Medical Association, American College of Physicians, American

College of Surgeons, and Canadian Hospital Association to certify the safety and quality of hospital performance. Accreditation standards included appropriate attention to medical staff organization, and trustees of accredited hospitals rarely considered that such things as unnecessary hospitalization or unnecessary surgery could occur in institutions anointed by the JCAH.

In 1966, the conditions for participation in Medicare required that every hospital must have a utilization review committee of the medical staff whose function was to review medical records systematically to make certain that admissions to the hospital were justifiable, length of stay was not excessive, and services rendered were appropriate. It was expected that the process would identify physicians whose practices were unsatisfactory, and, if their explanations were inadequate, the self-governing staff would take action to straighten out the offenders by educational and, if necessary, disciplinary measures. The system appeared to work well, with only the most flagrant cases of negligence or abuse calling for investigation and action by the board of trustees to terminate or curtail privileges.

The rising concern for effective utilization of hospital facilities and services that resulted in the utilization review provisions of Medicare had also brought about federal legislation in the 1960s creating comprehensive health service planning agencies and Regional Medical Programs, the first aimed at rationalizing the system by improved communitywide and areawide planning and the second seeking to encourage regionalization of communication and educational and consultative services so that innovations and improvements arising in the academic medical centers might be disseminated more readily through less favored institutions for the benefit of their constituencies.

The results in both cases were spotty. In some places, the availability of federal funding added resources and strength to already functioning voluntary health planning agencies; in others, and perhaps more, the imposition of federal requirements resulted in conflict and confusion. Health planning expertise was rare, and the condition of public representation on planning boards didn't by any means always result in decisions favoring the community as opposed to the medical profession and its institutions. There were instances, in fact, where hospital trustees serving on voluntary planning boards precisely in order to see that decisions were made in the interest of the whole community gave up and resigned when the public representation requirement was seen as giving the majority of positions on the boards to local politicians. Similarly, some Regional Medical Programs initiated useful and successful educational and consultative services, and some of these have continued, though many have petered out as federal funding was diminished over the years. In many areas, however, the

Regional Medical Program was feared by practitioners in smaller communities as a mechanism through which the academic medical centers would tell community physicians what to do, if not actually take over their patients, and in some cases these fears, at least in part, may have been justified.

Some of these problems have been resolved, or partially resolved, by more recent federal legislation, such as the Social Security Amendments of 1972 and the National Health Planning and Resources Development Act of 1974, and by the rise of the state regulatory authorities. But the new federal and state enactments have also created new problems for hospitals, as we shall see in later discussions. Whatever their effects have been, however, plainly the new entitlements and enactments have added another dimension to hospital function. In the 1960s and 1970s, all hospitals have become public health facilities—at least to the extent that some of their services are paid for by tax funds for patients who are public beneficiaries and to the extent that their activities are thus subject to regulation by public authority.

But it is a remarkable and perhaps unique characteristic of the hospital as a social organism that, unlike most others, it takes on new roles and responsibilities without discarding old ones. As we have seen, the hospital retained its function as charitable asylum when it became the doctor's workshop, and it has retained its functions as charitable asylum and doctor's workshop during the years it has also been a community medical enterprise, and unquestionably it will retain some of its functions as charitable asylum and doctor's workshop and community medical enterprise now that it is evolving also as public health facility. Unfortunately for the clarity with which the hospital is viewed by the community, by the public, and by the government, and even in some cases by physicians and hospital trustees themselves, however, the new roles and responsibilities are not laid on neatly, a layer at a time, and they cannot ever be clearly differentiated, one from another. The transitions instead are gradual, and often invisible, and so the functions are intermingled and interwoven and often inseparable, and the resulting image of the hospital may be as confusing as the pattern of a fabric woven by one who is color-blind. Some of the passive awe of the sick poor toward the charitable asylum remains, and to it has been added the grateful acceptance of the doctor's workshop by patients and families who were sometimes uneasy but always uncritical. This too remains, combining with the massive and often restive interest of the millions who have been paying their hospital bills by prepayment or insurance and see themselves as purchasers, or even partners, not beneficiaries. To this gallimaufry is added now the whole taxpaying population, rapidly being conditioned by its elected and appointed representatives in the Congress and the federal bureaus and the statehouses and legislatures and county councils and city halls to believe that whatever the names on the deeds and titles, the hospitals belong to them, and so they should have something to say about the plans, and the services, and the management, and the bills.

As often happens, these public representatives (and the group includes not just public officials but any number of union and corporation and Blue Cross and insurance executives and others who buy and bargain for health services on behalf of their members and employees and customers) commonly outrun their constituencies in the demands they make on the providers of health services. Thus they may criticize hospitals, for example, for shortcomings and failures the people they represent are not conscious of, and they may demand changes nobody else is especially aware of needing. Like the football fan who kept shouting from the stands, "Give the ball to Littlewood!" until the quarterback, exasperated, straightened up out of the huddle and shouted back, "Littlewood, he don't want the ball!" the surrogates keep on shouting their demands, and the understandable, exasperated response of some hospitals has been to shout back, sometimes overlooking the fact that the demands are not always bad, and that anyway some of the shouters are now paying customers, or even part owners, whose demands, good or bad, have to be taken seriously.

Some hospital trustees and physicians are infuriated by the shouting. When a community group publicly criticized a rich hospital for providing what was described as inadequate service for its community's black population, which was represented not at all on either the board or the medical staff and only sparsely in the patient population, a trustee castigated the group's spokesman. "What right has he got to criticize *us*?" the trustee fumed. "He's never even made a contribution to our building fund!" A physician at a city hospital complained bitterly about the time he was required to spend in the outpatient department, where, as he said, "These people come in off the streets and have to be seen, even when there's nothing the matter with them!"

Certainly it is understandable that trustees who contribute time and effort and money and worry to support their hospitals should be indignant when they get abuse instead of thanks for their pains, and that busy physicians should be frustrated when they must spend their time looking at sore throats and scratches in the outpatient department while their own offices may be filled with waiting patients who are both sicker and less demanding. But these are unavoidable facts of life in the public facility era. More and more trustees and physicians are recognizing that participation in the publicly funded programs, while it doesn't alter the hospital's status as a private corporation, is accompanied by an obligation to respond, or at least listen respectfully, to public demands, even when, as happens more often than not, they learn about the demands for the first time by means of a newspaper headline, not an orderly petition presented through channels.

Some of the demands are now enshrined in laws and regulations that foretell a time of rising pressure on trustees and physicians, and especially on administrators, who are often confronted with the unhappy, not to say impossible, task of explaining to physician A why the Social Security Administration has denied payment for his Medicare patient X and has approved payment for physician B's Medicare patient Y with the same diagnosis. Last week, the administrator had to explain to the trustees that the comprehensive health planning agency has turned down the hospital's application for a surgical specialty addition, which could have been expected to earn substantial revenues, with the suggestion that the hospital instead should expand its geriatric section, which is already a loser. Even more unsettling are the apparently whimsical administrative decisions that threaten hospital revenues—like the state authority's heavy-handed budget cuts or the sudden and not infrequent changes in the Medicare reimbursement formula. Invariably, the changes all lean in one direction, and the direction isn't up.

Added to these harassments are the strictures and demands that come from unofficial, but still public, sources: neighborhood and community groups of all kinds; old people, young people, black people, brown people; unions of nonprofessional workers who want more money for less work; and associations of professional employees, not excluding physicians, who want the same thing and don't hesitate to use the same tactics. The hospital is a target for them all; confrontation and negotiation are becoming the way of life in hospital management. Invariably, the trustees who only yesterday stood apart as fiduciaries, fund raisers, and policy formulators seem more and more to be drawn into the confrontations and negotiations. Traditionally, trustees are the bridge between the institution and the community; they still are, but the traffic on the bridge is getting heavier all the time.

Most of the new pressures and problems probably belong somewhere under the rubric "accountability." Of course, hospital trustees have always been accountable in a way to themselves, and in a way to the patients and families and communities their institutions serve, and in a way to the physicians who practice in the institutions and to the employees who work there, and in a way to their sources of funding and the licensing and public health authorities in whose jurisdictions they operate their institutions and programs. For the most part, however, these accountabilities have been more perfunctory than exacting. The trustee who didn't show up for meetings was more likely to be kidded for his dereliction than reprimanded or replaced. Until recently, patients and their families had only minor complaints; lawsuits were rare. Physicians got what they wanted. Philanthropists were either undemanding or got on the board and started running things. Licensing and public health authorities stayed in the woodwork and kept quiet.

Now all this has changed. The terms of all these accountabilities have been converted from what was more than anything else an agreeable obeisance to good form to what has become instead a nagging insistence on good performance. New parties to the accountability contract are springing out from behind the trees to present lists of their expectations and demands, with copies to the press and broadcast media. Hospital administrators, trustees, and physicians frequently complain that their institutions are unduly criticized, if not persecuted, by the press, but the fact is that the media are not so much the abusers as they are used by the abusers. Any politician seeking a headline, and all politicians seek headlines all the time, has only to take a shot at the nearest hospital with an allegation of excessive cost, or inefficiency, or slow service, or whatever, and the hospital is immediately on the defensive. If the newspaper or TV station is honest, and conscientious, and has time, it will call the hospital for a response. Most hospitals today are prepared with answers, but the disadvantage lingers. The charges are generally unprovable, and the answers are too complex for quick reporting and easy comprehension. A flat denial lacks credibility. The only constructive course hospitals have discovered is the long, painstaking public relations task of educating news people in hospital affairs to the point where they can distinguish between the phony, self-serving charge and the informed, honest criticism. When this is done, the hospital is more likely to get fair treatment, at least until the educated reporter moves on to another assignment and the process has to go back to the starting line. As natural spokesmen for their hospitals, trustees have many opportunities to answer the same charges, publicly as well as privately, but the evidence suggests that they are not invariably prepared for the task.

Difficult as they unquestionably are, all these new problems of management and regulatory authority and public expectation and demand are in territory that is familiar to many hospital trustees. Most of them have management problems in their own businesses or activities. Regulatory authority impinges on us all, if not elsewhere then certainly at income tax time, and the pervasive phenomena of unreal public expectations and demands are familiar to anyone who reads the news and watches television.

Another area of trustee responsibility that has also been changing rapidly in recent years, and is now considered by many trustees and many others to have superseded finance as the most important of all trustee functions, however, is accountability for the quality of medical service. Here the terrain is as unfamiliar and treacherous as finance is near and known. There are road maps showing the way to go, but only the knowledgeable and experienced know how to read the maps, and not even all of these are bold enough to push ahead or always make the right turnings.

Like the other areas, it has always been there, at least theoretically. But unlike the others, in the past it has been observed perfunctorily, if at all. It was the doctors' business to choose staff members with care for their credentials, to assign privileges, to keep an eye out for inevitable error and occasional malefaction, and to take appropriate action, with minimum visibility, and then make suitable reports and recommendations to the board as the ultimate repository of responsibility. There were occasions of conflict, to be sure, but they were rare. Some boards dared to prod when medical staffs failed to act in cases patently requiring discipline, but few had the stomach to pursue any dispute over the border onto the doctors' grounds. Even after the American College of Surgeons, the American Hospital Association, and the JCAH were declaring that medical quality *was* the board's responsibility, the territory was regarded as unsafe, and at best it was always uncomfortable.

This, too, has changed. In decisions going back to the early days of the JCAH, the courts had held consistently that private hospitals had the right and the duty to set standards of performance for physicians using their facilities. Customarily, the hospital delegated responsibility for maintaining the standards to the medical staff, and the staff bylaws spelled out the procedure for monitoring performance and dealing with deficiencies. If the bylaws comprehended due process and its provisions were strictly observed, the courts had little sympathy for doctors whose privileges were terminated or curtailed.

Then, interestingly, at about the time the Great Society legislation was ushering hospitals into the public-interest era, came a series of court decisions suggesting that the hospital, which is to say the board of trustees, has a duty that may go beyond delegation to the medical staff and backing up its recommendations. In the celebrated case of *Darling v. Charleston Community Memorial Hospital,* the jury ruled for the plaintiff patient and held the *hospital corporation* liable for not intervening through its employed administrator and nurses to prevent the damage that occurred because of the negligence of an attending physician. In denying an application for rehearing, the Supreme Court of Illinois, ruling in 1965, relied on an earlier New York decision that read in part: "The conception that the hospital does not undertake to treat the patient, does not undertake to act through its doctors and nurses, but undertakes instead simply to procure them to act upon their own responsibility, no longer reflects the fact. Present-day hospitals, as their manner of operation plainly demonstrates, do far more than furnish facilities for treatment. . . . The person who avails himself of hospital facilities expects that the hospital will attempt to cure him, not that its nurses or other employees will act on their own responsibility."[2]

As will be seen when these new accountabilities are examined in greater detail in later chapters, we've come a long way from the days of the charitable asylum and doctor's workshop.

3.

WHO'S
ON BOARDS?

The genus *hospital* as we know it today had its origin in the temples of healing of antiquity and the religious asylums of the Middle Ages, but the species *American voluntary* emerged directly from the marriage of medical knowledge or practice and philanthropic impulse. The mating occurred in different ways, according to circumstance. Often it was a skilled and ambitious surgeon who stirred the imagination of a millowner or landowner whose beneficence provided the foundation, if not the entire structure, of a hospital that grew with the community over the years, perpetuating the name of the founder, perhaps as a memorial to the surgeon or to the founder's family. In a surprising number of cases the spark was provided by the millowner's wife or widow, and in more than just one or two of those Annie L. Smith Memorial Hospitals, Annie turns out to have been the surgeon's dedicated nurse and, long before the term was invented, management consultant.

Whoever the originators were, they needed help, and, since the founders more often than not were no longer young, they needed supporters to carry on the purposes of the hospital after they were gone. These responsibilities were given over to trustees, whose original function was simply and solely to safeguard the property and thus protect the trust established by the founders. Then, as now, the preferred method of safeguarding was expanding, as an army defends by attacking, and so the trustees were chosen with a careful eye for their access to assets. The heirs to the mills, factories, and farms were natural choices; bankers and lawyers were obviously strategic additions. Property and links to property were the sought-for qualifications.

For all the variations in hospital origin and function that have evolved over the years, the selection of trustees hasn't changed that much. In several recent surveys conducted by or for the American Hospital Association, state hospital associations, management consultants, foundations, and others, including, in the aggregate, several thousand members of hospital boards of trustees, from half to two-thirds of all the trustees were found to be bankers, lawyers, or owners or managers of businesses. Understandably, the distribution of occupations changes with size of hospital and size of community, with the owners and managers of small businesses prevailing in the smaller communities, and corporate executives— what has come to be called the managerial class—predominating on the larger boards in the cities. In the smaller communities, too, there are more housewives, clergymen, and "others" among the trustees, and in the cities more investment bankers and "other professionals," a designation that includes university professors, industrial psychologists, and management consultants. But the old practice holds: In a survey of the occupations of board presidents or chairmen of teaching hospitals, 80 percent were executives, bankers, or lawyers. [1]

This is not to say that there have been no changes at all in the composition of hospital boards. One change has already emerged as a visible trend, and another is on the horizon and seems certain to advance rapidly under the pressure of external forces impinging on hospitals in the era of public funding.

The change that has already occurred is the lowering of the traditional barrier to membership of practicing physicians on hospital boards. The early origins of the tradition are not precisely clear; most likely, it was nothing more than the disposition of physicians to tell their benefactors, "You take care of the money, and we'll look after the patients," and the reciprocal disposition of owners and managers to consider that doctors are poor businessmen, which is not invariably the case.

As sometimes happens in business as well as hospitals, customary practice develops its own rationale, and the physician trustee who was at first only a departure from customary practice became in time a sin against the hospital culture. In a textbook first published in 1935 and long regarded as the bible of hospital management, Malcolm T. MacEachern, M.D., who was for years associate director of the American College of Surgeons and conducted its hospital standardization program, forerunner of the Joint Commission on Accreditation of

Hospitals, listed the reasons physicians shouldn't be elected to boards: Trusteeship would give the physician undue publicity and thus a competitive advantage over his colleagues; he would use the position for his own advantage and thus could not be considered a representative of the medical staff. In fact, board-staff relationships would deteriorate, not improve, because of the jealousy of other staff members, who would come to regard the physician trustee as an inspector or policeman for the board. Besides, the doctor on the board would have a conflict of interest, personal gain as against, institutional loyalty, if not actual double jeopardy because of his legal responsibility as trustee. Finally, the accepted method of reappointing physicians annually to membership on the medical staff would be weakened, and on occasion possibly embarrassed, when the physician trustee was required to vote on his own reappointment. "The practice is generally seen as undesirable," Dr. MacEachern concluded.[2] The way things turned out, that was stating the case conservatively.

Obviously, there had to be some systematic communication between the board and the medical staff. Throughout the American College of Surgeons years and into the era of the JCAH, the generally accepted vehicle was a joint conference committee with members representing both bodies, plus the administrator. The committee system appeared to work well for most purposes, but doctors sometimes complained that the joint conference committee couldn't decide anything. Difficult problems tended to disappear into board meetings, and doctors learned what happened only after action had been taken. As an equal partner with the AHA on the JCAH board, the American Medical Association began to press its representatives on the board to seek JCAH action making physician membership on hospital boards of trustees acceptable, if not mandatory.

The fact that some few hospitals had always had physician trustees was known but, like the alcoholic uncle in the family, never talked about, until the mid-1950s, when a joint AMA-AHA statement on hospital-physician relationships was presented to the AHA House of Delegates for approval. The statement named physician membership on the hospital board of trustees as one of several acceptable methods of board-staff communication and action. It was approved, finally, by the AHA delegates, but only after extended debate during which the traditionalists gave ground reluctantly. The testimony of hospitals that had physician trustees and found them helpful, not hurtful, wasn't disbelieved, actually, but many administrators had been conditioned to believe that conflict and jealousy had to be lurking there in the boardrooms, just waiting to be found out.

Twenty years later, in 1974, the issue was debated again in the AHA House of Delegates when a policy statement advocating physician membership on hospital boards was under consideration, and again the resistance was formidable, although by this time a few surveys indicated that as many as half the hospitals had at least one physician board member, and some had several, and the disastrous consequences feared by Dr. MacEachern had not ensued. Yet when a foundation study of the governance of teaching hospitals in New York City was reported to a meeting of board members of the participating institutions, the one among some two dozen recommendations that was singled out for heated debate was that the hospitals would be well advised to elect physicians to their boards.[3]

"Although there are other satisfactory ways of presenting medical information and opinion to hospital trustees," the Macy report said, "bringing doctors who have the whole institution as their interest to the same level of public accountability as other trustees will make for better governance." The Macy study, however, stopped short of recommending that physician trustees should be elected as representatives of the medical staff. "Experience indicates that they should not be elected by the medical staff to represent its interests on the board, the way an alderman votes for street improvements in his ward at city council meetings," the report said. "Rather, the physician trustees should be elected to membership in precisely the same way as the other trustees are elected. They should take part in board deliberations and decision-making in the interest of the whole hospital, and the mission and community it serves, and not as the representative of any constituency within the whole." In theory, at least, this seems to be a sound approach, but the more common practice has been for the elected president of the staff, and sometimes the vice-president and other officers, to sit on the board by virtue of their staff offices. Whatever the method of their selection, it would be hard for physicians practicing in the hospital to be on the board without representing the interests of the staff in some ways. A few hospitals have avoided the issue entirely by electing only physicians who are not members of the active staff. In most cases this has meant retired physicians, whose information and ideas may not always be up to date—a circumstance that may be an improvement over no physicians at all, but not much of an improvement.

The Macy report also recommended another change in board composition that is widely understood to be inevitable eventually but hasn't occurred yet, probably because the pressure hasn't developed sufficiently. "There has been a persistent clamor for neighborhood or community or consumer groups to have representation," the report said. "The most severe pressures have emerged in inner-city neighborhoods and communities. This occurs because such groups feel excluded from the mechanism of control, without a voice in having their needs met by the institution which is there to serve them." The need for such representation is valid, the report said, but the most effective method of meeting it may be the appointment of community committees to deal directly with management and staff on matters that concern them. Among the members of such committees, it was suggested, good trustee candidates may be identified who can then be elected to the board and "bring to the trusteeships a dimension that has often been missing: a thoughtful understanding of patient and community needs and feelings and a willingness to listen and learn about the hospital's resources and limitations. It should be understood, however, that the self-surfacing or self-elected neighborhood leader who brings only demands and not the willingness to listen will be a burden, and not an asset, to the governing process. Like the physician trustee, the board member who is present as a user of hospital services can illuminate deliberations by his understanding of patient, family, and neighborhood response to the hospital and its services, but he can contribute to board decisions only if he comprehends the whole institution."

Consumer representation on hospital boards is not a new concept. The early gospel according to MacEachern declared that "Board members should be representative citizens. All sections of the community should have representation: the learned professions, business interests, organized labor, women's clubs all should be represented either directly or indirectly."

Later, in 1946, the report of a prestigious national Commission on Hospital Care, whose membership included such illustrious citizens as former President Herbert Hoover, Secretary of the Army Thomas Gates, and General Motors executive Charles S. Kettering, urged that hospital trustees should be "broadly representative of the public served by the institution. Representatives of agriculture, industry, labor, and other groups of consumers of hospital services should be included in the membership. In some instances it may be desirable and helpful to include representatives from local government. The policies they formulate should reflect the needs and desires of the public. It is essential that they should regard their position as one of public duty and responsibility rather than one of preference and honor."[4]

With so many authorities making so many recommendations over so many years, one might think that by this time the hospital boardroom would resemble a town meeting, but of course that isn't what has happened at all. With a few exceptions, mostly in the inner-city hospitals in deprived neighborhoods, boards look pretty much the same today as they did a generation ago and have looked, in fact, for several generations—with the single exception, as we have seen, of the addition of physician members.

Challenged about "consumer representation," most board members insist that they are "consumers" and their boards are representative of their communities. "Who could be more representative than these men and women?" a board chairman might ask a visitor, beaming down the table at the assembled bankers,

lawyers, merchants, and auxiliary leaders, and of course they *are* representative—
though possibly only in the sense that Louis XV was representative of 18th-
century France.

In the cities, board members are more troubled than puzzled by the question.
They understand that in the modern sense "consumer" means something more
than "nonprofessional." It refers, instead, to all those who have no role at all in
the provision of services, as most trustees certainly do have, and in most contexts
it refers particularly to the groups that have been unrepresented in the past not just
on hospital boards but in community and public affairs generally. There are some
hospital board members still, and some physicians, who deny that such groups
need or should have any voice at all in planning or shaping the services provided
for them: "What do they know about it?" is the attitude that can still be observed.
But there are more who are willing to concede that people receiving services paid
for in part by public funds should have something to say about what the services
are.

How are the consumer representatives to be selected? And wouldn't they make
board meetings awkward, and board decisions difficult to arrive at? How would it
work? "I know we're going to have to bring some neighborhood people in here
some time, probably before long," the administrator of a teaching hospital told a
reporter who asked about community representatives. "But what am I supposed
to do? Go out in the street and buttonhole somebody going by? And what will
happen then? Our board members now all know each other and are used to
working together effectively, and they have done great things here, including
great things *for the neighborhood!* I suppose this will have to change some day, but
I'm afraid it may be worse, not better, because of the change."

Not necessarily. These are understandable misgivings, but the fact is that there
are tested methods of selecting and working with neighborhood leaders, as the
Macy report suggested, and, although city hospitals have had some problems
getting such mechanisms as community advisory committees to work, most of
them acknowledge that they have learned from the experience and that services
have been improved as a result. A lot of city hospital drug abuse and alcohol
services, departments of community medicine, youth centers, and ombudsman or
patient representative programs started life as shouting matches. It isn't the
method anybody in his right mind would choose, perhaps, but it isn't impossible,
and it may be preferable to becoming an island in a neighborhood that grows
increasingly restive.

Meanwhile, there are other problems suggesting that the long-standing
methods of choosing hospital board members may have to be reexamined. An
aging member of a New York law firm explained how the system has worked. "We

ask our friends in the banks and investment houses and law firms who the younger men are who will be taking over in a few years," he said. "Then we get to know them, if we don't already, by asking for their help with a hospital fund-raising project, or their advice on some problem in their field. Then, when the time comes, we nominate them for trusteeship. They always accept." A younger board member of another hospital described the same process from another perspective. How did you get on the board? he was asked. "My boss told me to," he replied.

The bosses and the bright young men may have to pause and consider some new questions that have been arising in recent years. Following disclosure by a Washington newspaper that several hospitals in the District of Columbia maintained large deposits in banks whose officers were trustees of the hospitals, one of the institutions was sued on behalf of a group of citizens who charged that the trustees had conspired for their own personal gain at the expense of the hospital's patients, who were required to pay costs that were elevated unnecessarily as a result of the trustees' actions. The U.S. District Court in which the case was tried found no evidence of conspiracy and no evidence of any personal gain or aggrandizement on the part of any of the trustees concerned. However, the court did find that the hospital had maintained substantial sums in savings and checking accounts rather than in Treasury bonds or investments, and the court concluded that the defendant trustees had breached their fiduciary duty to supervise the management of the hospital's investments. The court then ordered that each trustee should disclose in writing to the full board of trustees "his or her affiliations, if any, with any bank, savings and loan association, investment firm or other financial institution presently doing business with the hospital" and must thereafter amend the written report quarterly to reflect any changes. The court also ordered that the hospital's auditors must incorporate into each annual audit a written summary of all business conducted during the preceding fiscal year between the hospital and any bank, savings and loan association, investment firm, or other financial institution with which any hospital officer or trustee is affiliated as a trustee, director, partner, general manager, principal officer, or substantial stockholder, and must make a copy of the audit reports available on request for inspection by any patient of the hospital at the hospital's offices during business hours.[5]

Because of the Washington episode and similar conflict-of-interest disclosures involving hospital trustees elsewhere, members of Congress have suggested legislation that would make it mandatory for hospitals participating in Medicare, Medicaid, and other federally funded programs to make public statements of the financial interests and connections of trustees, including information about trustee interest in any firms doing any business with the hospital and evidence that goods or services were purchased by the hospital from such firms only on the basis of competitive bids. Similar written disclosure of any possible conflict of interest by hospital trustees, officers, and employees with administrative responsibilities has also been recommended for its member hospitals by the American Hospital Association, and the subject was recently examined in detail in a study conducted by the General Accounting Office of the United States.[6]

In a report to the Congress, the GAO said its review of arrangements between hospitals and members of their governing and advisory boards and key employees had been conducted to determine what kind of information would be made public if a disclosure requirement were to be included in legislation. The GAO study also examined the arrangements between hospitals and hospital-based specialists (pathologists and radiologists).

Because the overlapping interests of hospital governing board members or key employees may detrimentally affect hospital costs and general administration, the GAO report noted, it has been suggested that all such arrangements should be made public. Outright conflicts of interest are either prohibited or required to be disclosed in corporate statutes in many of the states, but in view of the interest of the Congress, the courts, the news media, and the general public it seemed appropriate to look at the issue of public accountability in public and quasi-public organizations—that is, hospitals. The GAO considered that an "overlapping interest" was "the holding by a hospital board member or employee of a position or of a financial interest in any concern (1) from which a hospital secures goods or services or (2) which competes with the hospital for the delivery of medical care. A hospital board member or employee who provides consulting or other services to any outside concern doing business with the hospital is also considered to have an overlapping interest."

The GAO study reviewed such interests as they were found to exist in 19 hospitals located in the metropolitan Washington, DC, area and in Kansas City, St. Louis, and Springfield, MO. "We did not attempt to evaluate the propriety or reasonableness of a particular overlapping arrangement," the report said. "We have identified and described the type of information that would be publicly disclosed were a disclosure requirement established." Arrangements involving overlapping interests were found at 17 of the 19 hospitals, the GAO said. "Our review of 19 hospitals was not intended to be representative of all hospitals in the country. However, since business and professional leaders typically serve on boards of nonprofit organizations, we believe that review of additional hospitals in other areas would show that the existence of overlapping interests was not unusual," the report added.

The type and extent of overlapping interests that were found varied from hospital to hospital, it was reported, but the one that occurred most often was the association of members of the governing or advisory boards with banks or investment or legal firms. "Some of these relationships probably benefitted the hospitals by fostering favorable loans and expert management of hospital assets," the GAO report said. In another commonly occurring overlap, members of governing boards included officials of local newspapers or public utilities with which the hospital necessarily did business. "The boards of the nonprofit hospitals we reviewed generally were composed of community business leaders who had expressed an interest in the hospital's welfare," said the report. "The hospitals' nomination and election procedures varied, as did the professional background of board members. Most hospitals judged each nominee's background individually and did not possess specific criteria for board qualification. At the [one] profit-making hospital we reviewed, the board was generally composed of medical staff members who brought with them substantial patient business."

At all the hospitals that were reviewed in the Washington area there was evidence that the governing boards had considered the overlapping relationships and were aware of the problems that might arise if the relationships were not disclosed, the GAO indicated. "However, only two of the six [Washington] boards had passed resolutions requesting board members to submit replies to questionnaires disclosing overlapping relationships to an executive committee of the board." Board members at both these hospitals had complied with the request, it was reported. "GAO found little evidence that these arrangements increased hospital costs," the report said. "In fact, they may have been beneficial. In some cases, individuals or their companies made donations to the hospitals far exceeding any financial gains that could have been realized from such arrangements."

As a result of its investigation, the GAO concluded that any attempts to prohibit overlapping interests would be impractical. However, it added, "We believe that public confidence in these institutions would be enhanced if the issue of overlapping interests were faced openly through public disclosure, including a statement of the extent of competition involved in acquiring goods and services." The GAO recommended that the Congress should consider amending the Social Security Act to require that such disclosure be made a condition for participating in Medicare, Medicaid, and Maternal and Child Health and Crippled Children's Services and that such a provision should also be considered for inclusion in any national health insurance program legislation.

The American Hospital Association and the American Medical Association disagree. Commenting on the GAO report and recommendation, the AHA said the issues it raised are important but can be handled adequately through internal disclosure requirements such as those recommended for its member institutions by

AHA and through other processes already carried out by most health care institutions in meeting their public trust and responsibilities. Disclosure require-ments in existing legislation and regulations can deal with the issue successfully, the AHA concluded; additional legislation such as that proposed by GAO is neither necessary nor justified. Agreeing that the legislation is unnecessary, the AMA argued that the public would be confused and perhaps misled by such information and that the broad publicity and concern for overlapping interest or potential conflicts of interest would discourage highly qualified individuals from serving on hospital boards.[7]

That could happen, but it isn't seen as a serious problem by a man whose experience as a banker, public official, and trustee may readily exceed that of most entire boards. This is Joseph W. Barr, chairman of the board of directors of the American Security and Trust Company, one of the banks whose officers were involved in the Washington, DC, hospital conflict-of-interest disclosure by the *Washington Post* a few years ago. Mr. Barr has also been a member of Congress, Secretary of the Treasury of the United States, chairman of the Federal Deposit Insurance Corporation, and director or trustee of a number of corporations and nonprofit organizations. As a banker, he dismissed out of hand the charge that officers of his own and other Washington banks were guilty of conflicts of interest because the hospitals they served as trustees kept large demand deposits in their banks. "Frankly, I thought the money charge was crazy," he said. "In my lifetime I have seen too many individuals and too many organizations get into difficulties because they have engaged in overly sophisticated cash management to alter my admittedly conservative approach to cash balances."[8]

Nevertheless, Mr. Barr acknowledged, the issue is a serious one, for the Washington banks and for all banks and institutions. "It has long been a practice for nonprofit organizations such as hospitals to include bankers on their boards either as trustees or directors," he said in an address to a regional institute on bank administration not long after the conflict-of-interest episode erupted in Washington. "In an area such as medical care, where the costs are becoming increasingly onerous, it is only natural that public attention will be focused sharply on the management of these institutions. Therefore, we seem to be faced with a dilemma. We can permit our officers to serve as trustees of nonprofit organizations with the knowledge that we may be exposing our banks to conflict-of-interest charges. Or we can decline to serve on these boards and refuse to accept any responsibility for their management. One might argue that the proper course is to accept our community responsibilities, to serve on the boards, and to make sure that no conflict-of-interest situations arise. Frankly, I doubt that this is possible. Prudent men can arrive at decisions which to them bear no taint of conflict of interest but which appear very differently to newspaper reporters, politicians, and the general public. I conclude that there is no easy answer."

After relating a number of conflicts he had encountered in government and private business, Mr. Barr said he had often argued with the officers of his bank that they were granting unduly low loan rates to the nonprofit organizations they supported. "They argue that these organizations deserve the prime rate," he reported. "I argue that rarely if ever do these nonprofit groups meet the credit standards of a prime rate customer; the nonprofit organizations should be supported by corporate giving rather than through cut-rate business transactions. It may be that shareholders rather than nonprofit groups suffer from close affiliations."

On balance, Mr. Barr concluded, he did not intend to pull his officers back from their civic obligations. "I have warned them that they must be increasingly careful of conflict-of-interest situations. But I am certain that in the future as they discharge their obligation to these nonprofit institutions they may well take actions which to an outsider seem to smack of conflict of interest. I am certain that in the future we will be subjected to further attacks by the press or the Congress. But the neglect of our civic institutions is a much more serious subject than the occasional criticism we may receive. Therefore, I offer this advice: Fulfill your civic obligations. Take care of the nonprofit organizations, watch out for conflicts of interest, realize that public criticism is inevitable, and keep your fingers crossed that the criticism will not unduly tarnish our reputations or drop our price-earnings multiples."

If Mr. Barr's advice is sound for bankers, it would appear to apply as well for lawyers, physicians, brokers, investment and management consultants, insurance agents, merchants, manufacturers, public utilities executives, and others who are serving on hospital boards today, and also, with appropriate accommodation for organizational objectives other than price-earning multiples, for the neighborhood, community, and other consumer representatives who are certain to become hospital trustees in the years ahead. Conflicts of interest are by no means a monopoly of the business community, and the possibility that consumer trustees could favor their outside organizational objectives as opposed to the hospital's has to be considered.

One consumer organization, for example, Ralph Nader's Health Research Group, has declared among its objectives the public dissemination of such information as infection rates, use of antibiotics and other drugs, tissue committee reports, physician profiles, and other data most hospitals would consider highly confidential and subject to harmful misinterpretation. In fact, the Joint Commission on Accreditation of Hospitals releases information obtained during its surveys only to the hospitals themselves and recently sued the Department of Health, Education, and Welfare (HEW) for making public JCAH data turned over to the Social Security Administration in connection with a Medicare investigation. It can be argued, as the Health Research Group has done, that public accountability demands public disclosure, and it may be that hospital boards and medical staffs have been overly fearful of the harmful results of disclosure. But determination of information policy within the law must be left to the individual institution's board of trustees; if a decision is made to keep records confidential, the consumer trustee is obliged to abide by it, however much he may disagree. As is the case of the businessman who wants to sell his oil or insurance or whatever to the hospital, some such conflicts of interest are probably unavoidable, but everybody is better off when they are foreseen and resolved in advance. The consumer who can't live comfortably with an established policy of confidentiality, and can't change it, had better not be elected to the board.

Who decides who shall be elected to boards? In the past, the method has often been the one described by the New York lawyer: He and his fellow trustees selected colleagues, or colleagues of colleagues, who had exhibited qualities of competence and leadership of promising dimensions. The board was thus in effect self-elected and self-perpetuating, and among some 80 percent of voluntary nonprofit hospitals this is basically the method that still prevails,[9] though in about half of these the corporate structure of the nonprofit association stipulates that trustees or directors shall be elected by the association membership, usually an amorphous body of a hundred or more citizens who pay nominal dues and come to a membership meeting once a year to listen to a stylized annual report and routinely elect the slate of officers and trustees or directors presented by the nominating committee. Only rarely does such a membership organization reject a board candidate, and then it is usually under the pressure of a hot issue related to local politics, land use, or funding.

When the hospital is owned by a religious or fraternal or other group whose membership is not solely concerned with the hospital, the election of directors may be less of a formality. In some church organizations, for example, the hospital trustees may be appointed or elected by a hierarchical official or body representing the owners, and of course the directors of investor-owned and government-owned hospitals are also selected in one way or another by the owners or owning agency, such as a county commission or township board of supervisors.

Generally speaking, boards of profit-making and government hospitals have fewer members than those of nonprofit institutions, and in the latter group church-affiliated boards are smaller than nonprofit association boards. Size of hospital is also a determinant of board size. An AHA survey found hospitals with fewer than 100 beds had an average of 9 to 10 board members; 100-bed to 499-bed hospitals had 16 board members, on the average; and those with 500 or more beds had 22.[10] However, the variations and aberrations are abundant. Many hospitals have boards of trustees with 50 to 75 members, and one not-for-profit hospital in New York State reported recently to the Council of Teaching Hospitals of the Association of American Medical Colleges that its board had 187 members! Obviously in any such case the board of trustees is, in effect, the membership association, and real governing authority is vested in a small, manageable executive or management committee.

Whereas some authorities, including the American College of Hospital Administrators, have recommended limiting governing board size in the interest of better management, others have seen no particular harm in large boards, so long as the members understand their legal responsibilities as trustees and are informed and satisfied with the performance of the effective governing or management group. "There can be no prescriptive size or composition for a hospital board of trustees," said Russell A. Nelson, M.D., in his report for the Macy Foundation. "The need is for men and women who are able, energetic, knowledgeable, and engaged. There is more danger of boards being too small than too large. Hospitals are in public business, and their trustees must be responsive and accountable to the public. Such a board certainly will include the leaders of business and industry, philanthropists and professionals who have been hospital trustees in the past, but it seems likely that others might be included who have not generally been represented on hospital boards, that is, women, young people, and outstanding individuals from minority racial, religious, or ethnic groups."

The terms of office for which trustees are elected or appointed also vary with ownership of the hospital. Directors of profit-making hospitals are commonly elected annually; government hospital board members usually have terms of one to three years; church and not-for-profit institutions report that terms of two, three, and sometimes four years are customary.

Most trustees are reelected at least once unless they have consistently failed to show up for meetings or otherwise indicated lack of interest, so the average duration in office runs from five to seven or eight years. Corporate bylaws sometimes limit the tenure of any trustee to two or three terms of office, thus preventing the awkwardness of having to find some acceptable way to get rid of a member who hasn't been effective but likes being a hospital trustee and isn't likely to withdraw voluntarily.

Some boards have amended their bylaws to add an age limitation, usually 70 or

75 years, to preclude the embarrassing and potentially damaging circumstance of an officer or trustee taking part in hospital decisions without an adequate grasp of what is going on.

Under today's conditions, an adequate grasp of what is going on isn't easy to achieve at any age, and awareness that this is the case is making boards more and more painstaking in examining the qualifications of nominees. The right business connections, reputation, and general visibility were adequate qualifiers for the less exacting responsibilities of a few years ago, but with state legislatures and the Congress and government bureaus and unions and consumer organizations and professional associations and the press and the public all looking critically at hospital decisions and hospital performance, the penalties for error are increasing, and the process of selection of trustees is becoming more rigorous accordingly.

"My first recommendation for serving on a hospital board is that all board members should expect to spend a substantial amount of time—and I am speaking of years—working on various committees to gain a practical understanding of how the institution runs," said James M. Underwood, former president of the Latrobe (PA) Hospital and a board member with a lot of mileage to his credit. [11] "To put it another way, board members should all be persons who have elected to make their hospital trusteeship a second long-term career. A hospital is too big, too complex, too vital to the community to afford any but working members on its policy-making body. There is no place for honorary members today."

In a recent publication, the Catholic Hospital Association specified the personal and professional qualifications that are desirable for board membership. Included among the personal qualifications were a commitment to community health and welfare and "translatable experience," or demonstrated managerial, technical, or professional experience providing evidence that the duties of hospital trusteeship can be performed effectively. Professional qualifications listed were technical competency in hospital or related health care enterprise, managerial competency, or knowledge and competence in educational, financial, legal, engineering, or other relevant professional fields. "The wise board, although constantly seeking to obtain the necessary competencies by appointing board members who possess them, will realize its own limitations and know when to seek outside counsel," the CHA publication concluded. [12]

It is in the nature of things that the counsel needed most often by the board is that of its own management, the hospital's administrator or chief executive officer, and increasingly today this fact is recognized by making the administrator a voting member of the board, usually with the title of president, instead of its servant or technical expert. Some administrators don't want to be board members, preferring the more removed role of agent with delegated authority, and some boards still prefer to delegate rather than share their authority with the chief executive. But the practice has become common and seems certain to continue to grow with the growing complexity of hospital operation. "It seems plain that there can be only one proper solution for the confusion of authority and consequent lack of control which results when a misunderstanding exists about who is in charge of the institution," said Dr. Nelson in the Macy report. "There must be an explicitly identified, full-time, salaried chief executive, visibly vested with full responsibility for the total enterprise and accountable to the board of trustees for fulfillment of its mission. The most appropriate title for the chief executive officer is president. He should be a voting member of the board of trustees, whose presiding officer would then logically be designated its chairman."

The principal objections to this so-called corporate form of organization for the voluntary hospital have come from those who consider it somehow invading the autonomy or independence of the medical staff, which traditionally has seen itself as a self-governing body responsible ultimately to the board but only indirectly within the jurisdiction of the management. These relationships are examined in greater detail in chapter 6, but the fact is that it is the outside world, not the internal organization, that has threatened or impinged on the independence of the medical staff. The government, the courts, and the public consider the hospital and its medical staff indistinguishable, however they may see themselves, and thus it has seemed sensible if not essential for the visible organizational structure to reflect the real world. Whatever way the board, administration, and staff may wish to define their relationships internally, nobody else views them as anything but a single entity. It is called the hospital, and unless it can be an entity, as well as being viewed as one, it might not survive the pressures of our time.

4. WHAT BOARDS DO: HOW THEY WORK

As laws and regulations affecting what hospitals do and how it should be done have multiplied in recent years, a few observers have suggested that the time may be coming when boards of trustees as we have known them in the past may no longer be needed. With the new planning agencies telling us what we can and can't do, and government reimbursement policies determining how much we'll be paid, and what for, there won't be much left for trustees to decide, in this view. Certainly it is true, at least, that trustees have less latitude today for determining institutional policy and directing institutional operations than they had in the past, and it may be true also that the area of independent action will diminish further over time as government funding increases, as it seems likely to do. But as the areas for decision and action may be shrinking on one dimension they are expanding on another as new technology, new needs and demands for services, and new organizational concepts are developing, and the prevailing opinion among members of Congress, public officials, and hospital leaders in the private sector, including trustees, is that in the era of public funding trustee responsibility is increasing, not diminishing.

The very fact that functions and values in the health care system are changing so rapidly intensifies the need for trustees whose dedication to the hospital and its goals is unquestioned but whose judgment, somewhat removed from the turbulent center of operations, is less likely to be affected by the pressures of immediate circumstance. In times of stress, especially, the "sounding board" function of trustees—the place where ideas and answers are tested—can be invaluable to administrators and physicians. It works both ways, as a stimulus or prod to professionals who are inclined to be fearful of change and cling to familiar methods and as a brake on those who would leap to embrace every new concept that comes along. As Professor Karl Weintraub of the University of Chicago once remarked in response to a challenge for reform in the universities, "With all respect for our love of change, we need angry old men willing to protect some of the olive trees painstakingly planted by former generations."

Now this is not to suggest that hospital trustees are, or should be, or ever have been, angry old men, and, in fact, the disposition of boards everywhere has been to meet the new problems and oncoming forces by recruiting younger men and women for trusteeship responsibility. In spite of the formidably increasing responsibilities, not excluding personal liability, that have often been mentioned as barriers to recruitment of new trustees, capable young people who are willing to take on the assignment are coming forward all the time. Given the heavy weight of tradition pointing to the election of trustees who have already arrived at positions of eminence in their chosen occupations, it is remarkable that nearly a third of the respondents in a recent nationwide survey of hospital trustees were men and women in their thirties or forties. It is plain that hospital boards are going to have their share of challengers daring to uproot the olive trees as well as protectors resolved to preserve them.

The American Hospital Association, Catholic Hospital Association, state hospital associations, regional and metropolitan hospital councils, and other groups in their publications have all listed the responsibilities and functions of hospital boards of trustees: establishing goals and policies; planning facilities and services; making provision for the organizational and financial resources needed to carry out institutional purposes; weighing and balancing the always divergent and sometimes contradictory demands of patients, physicians, employees, third parties, government officials, neighbors, and that ever-present plexus of interests and forces that we call the public. However they may be enumerated, board responsibilities all relate in one way or another to money, management, or medicine, and the purpose of this account is not to add another prescription to the already abundant literature but to report how trustees are responding in these areas to the problems and forces arising in our time.

One way they are responding is by working harder. Boards and committees meet oftener and longer than they used to do, taking more time and talk to resolve problems and reach decisions. At a recent regional meeting where trustees from a number of hospitals were exchanging experiences, one of them said, "You put all these things together—regulation, threats of lawsuit, problems in administration, and association of a lay board with medical people—and you may suddenly tell yourself, 'I'm having more fun than I can stand!' " Everybody laughed, and there was general agreement that the job had turned out to be more demanding, and often more frustrating, than had been foreseen. But nobody would say he wouldn't have accepted the appointment if he had known all that was going to be involved, and nobody was planning to resign.

A survey conducted by the AHA's magazine *Trustee* suggested the reason. Asked why they had agreed to become trustees, nearly all those questioned gave the ritual responses about opportunity to "serve the community" and "help people."[1] Next to these, the two most frequent reasons mentioned were the challenging responsibility and the desire to improve the way the hospital was being run. For such people, the fact that the challenge is in Macy's window unquestionably adds to the attraction. Only 8 percent of the survey respondents mentioned prestige as a factor influencing acceptance, but the public visibility of hospital trusteeship is not to be either discounted or derogated as a reason strong people are willing to take on, and stay on, a tough job. The man who was having more fun than he could stand probably wouldn't stand for it anyplace else.

Plainly, then, the traditional, fiduciary role of safeguarding the property and purpose for which the trust was created remains, but to it there has been added the more demanding duty to cope with the forces of change. Obviously, however, not all boards are busy all the time. In some communities still, some trustees are content to fill the traditional role and let administrators and physicians bear the brunt of change. But even where this is the case there is some awareness of the laws and regulations and court decisions that make trustees more accountable than they have been in the past, and it is doubtful that there can be a hospital board anywhere today that hasn't one or two members, at least, who have become better informed and more active than the busiest trustees were a generation ago in those easier, "we'll get the money and you run the place" days.

Usually these super trustees, the better informed and more active ones, have been trustees of their hospitals for years, serving terms as members and chairmen of planning and finance and professional relations committees and then, as officers and members of executive committees, becoming the real shapers of policies and decisions. In some cases the super board may be a single trustee; in other institutions there may be a group of three or four or half a dozen super trustees who share the information and the power and pass it on eventually to those they select as their successors. Sometimes these super board members have been reluctant about sharing information and authority with other members of their boards. Only rarely is this because they consciously want to keep all the power to themselves; more often it is simply a matter of efficiency as they see it. They know what needs to be done and how to work with the executive and medical staffs to get it done, and they doubt that anyone else could do it as well as they can.

Now this is a somewhat oversimplified account of how boards work, and obviously it is more true of some boards than of others. Yet a reporter who has been an observer of hospital practice for years and has attended board meetings and conferences and interviewed and conversed with trustees of all kinds and sizes of hospitals in all kinds and sizes of communities has found only a few instances in which the variation from this pattern was anything more than a matter of degree.

Sometimes the super board member, or one of them, is a physician who may or may not be a trustee himself. More and more often in recent years the hospital administrator is either *the* super board member or one of the inner group, again in some cases without actually being a trustee. It isn't often true, however, as it is commonly supposed, that the super board member is an executive or capitalist who has retired and works for the hospital because he has nothing else to do. Follow one of them around for a few days, or talk to him (or, rarely but not unexceptionally, her) for more than a few minutes, and you're pretty sure to find him in the same role in his own business, or businesses, or law practice, and very likely in other affairs as well. Wherever they may be found, leaders are found leading. It shouldn't surprise anybody that this is the way hospitals are run, because the same matrix of power can be discovered in nearly all organizations. This is the way boards of regents of universities operate, and school boards, and corporate boards of directors, government bureaus, legislative assemblies, and associations, and it has been that way ever since Socrates got put away for criticizing the elders of ancient Greece.

In a hospital or elsewhere in human affairs, this basic pattern of governance is not likely to be overthrown or turned around, or, if that should happen, as it might in a merger or change of ownership, the pattern will be reestablished over time. But it is being modified in many, if not most, hospitals today, for several reasons.

The most obvious reason is simply that there is too much that has to be known and decided today for any one person or small group to retain all the information and power for itself. Hospital decisions require command of an extraordinary range of financial, technical, legal, medical, statutory, regulatory, and logistic data such as to defy comprehension by any person or group, and where decision makers must lean on staffs of experts, power is necessarily diluted. The super trustee who seeks nobody's counsel but his own would have to be an egomaniac today, and wrong decisions would quickly catch him up and compel some distribution of his authority. With reasonable prudence, super board members have to make certain that the board and management are adequately backed up with specialists in all these fields, and the specialists thus inevitably share some of the responsibility for decisions.

Trustees don't have to go far out of their way to find out what can happen when they permit super board members to keep all the cards. In the celebrated case of the Cedars of Lebanon Hospital of Miami, for example, a super board member, the hospital president, was found guilty of fraud and went to jail following disclosure of multimillion dollar financial jiggery-pokery that came to light when the hospital was in default of payments on a government loan. The other trustees didn't know what was going on. Nobody else went to jail, but the board members were not cast in the role of public benefactors when the story was unfolding day after day on page one of the Miami newspapers. In the conflict-of-interest case involving the Washington, DC, hospital (see chapter 3), where the trustees were considered by the court to have breached their fiduciary duty to the hospital, the judge emphasized that the hospital's board of trustees had a financial committee and an investment committee, but that actually financial management had been conducted by the hospital administrator and treasurer and that neither committee had even met for a matter of years. The trustees in this case suffered nothing more than embarrassing publicity and a court order requiring them to mend their ways, but here, clearly, was a demonstration that the super board method had proved inadequate for the demands of our time.

As will be seen later, a succession of new statutory and regulatory requirements, court decisions, and professional recommendations has emerged defining trustee responsibility for the quality of patient care. Trustees who make any attempt at all to keep abreast of what's going on, as most of them do, can't fail to understand that they had better know what the super board members are doing and deciding, and why, because they are all going to be held responsible for the consequences. More and more, trustees are demanding not just to be let in on the secrets but to take part in the decisions, and super board members are agreeing not just that this is a good idea but that it's an absolute necessity. The super board will always be around, because that's the way things work, but it won't be as super as it used to be.

The model repository of trustee power is an executive committee authorized to act for the board when it is not in session and thus, in effect, a statutory super board that can be a legal and effective instrument of control. Executive committees may have as few as three or four members. In hospitals whose corporate formula calls for boards of trustees with 50 or more members, as some do, the executive committee may have 20 or 25 members; in these cases it is customary for the full board to meet only three or four times a year, and the executive committee meets monthly to conduct the hospital's business. Inevitably, then, the executive committee will have a super board of its own that provides continuity and either does everything that needs to be done or makes the machinery work.

On nearly all boards, the machinery is a structure of functional standing committees presumably having delegated authority to conduct studies, assemble data, formulate plans, and recommend action within their jurisdictions. In addition to board members appointed by the president or chairman, the standing committees may also include representatives of the administrative or medical staffs or other personnel, as appropriate. A typical hospital bylaw describes how the system works.

"Standing committees of the Board of Trustees are the primary working units of the Executive Committee. They review all matters falling within their areas of authority and discretion, including board policy decisions, budgets, major expenditures not included in the approved budgets, and monitoring hospital activities. The recommendations of the Standing Committees are forwarded to the Executive Committee for approval or disapproval. The meeting agenda for the committee will be developed jointly by the Committee Chairman and the President of the hospital. The minutes will record recommendations forwarded to the Executive Committee."

In addition to the executive committee, the functional committees found on most hospital organization charts include planning, finance, plant or property, personnel or labor relations, professional relations, and public or community relations. Other committees, standing or temporary, may deal with bylaws, nominations, investments, patient care, purchasing, real estate, legal problems, government relations, and liaison with other health agencies and institutions; in teaching hospitals there may be standing committees of the board on house staff, nursing, and medical education. Often there is a fund-raising committee whose function is distinguished from finance and investments, and a joint conference committee, including representatives of the board, administration, and medical staff, in addition to or in place of the professional relations committee.

The committee system makes perfectly good sense. The jurisdictions are de-fined areas of board responsibility. In some cases, as in fund-raising or legal problems, the board committee may actually conduct the hospital business or program; in others, as the bylaws specify, the committees recommend policies and control methods for consideration by the executive committee and, working with or through the administration, provide assistance, as needed, for general over-sight and solving problems. In practice, however, the system doesn't always work the way it should. Probably the most common reason it doesn't work, when it doesn't, is too many committees with not enough to do, and a few with too much. What happens then is that some committees either don't meet at all, or perhaps the members caucus for a few minutes before each board meeting so the chairman can report that "the committee met and reviewed current operations, which were judged satisfactory." The overworked members of the finance or government or public relations committee, in contrast, may find that they can't keep up with all the problems, and some of them by default are being handled by the administration, the executive committee, or the super board.

Though most of them are too polite, or too politic, to say so, most hospital administrators like it the way it is, and not the way it's supposed to be—a circumstance that has a lot to do with the fact that the two are not always the same. With a big board of trustees having a dozen or more committees that meet regularly, the administrator who spends most of his days and evenings in meetings anyway would have to choose between going to meetings around the clock and not knowing what his board was up to; not many hospitals have management staffs of the size and caliber that would be required to furnish effective executive assistance to a full complement of active board committees. A difference between the way the organization chart reads and the way the machinery of governance really works is unimportant in most cases, as long as the trustees know the controls are in place and operating effectively—a requirement that can be satisfied by an adequate system for detailed reporting of financial, management, and patient care activities. A trustee who spends his time reading reports may be performing his whole duty to the hospital, provided that he understands what they mean and has the wit and the will to blow the whistle when the figures don't look right.

Asked how he would describe the difference between management in business and management in the hospital, a man who had been instrumental in developing several successful businesses and had recently become a hospital trustee replied, "I can tell you in three words: control, control, control." As it happened, he hadn't been around hospitals long enough to understand that the chief difference in control lies in the unique latitude necessarily accorded to the medical staff, but the emphasis is impressive nevertheless.

The board committee structure may be either an instrument of control or an impediment to control, depending on how sensibly it is organized in relation to the nature and severity of the hospital's problems and on how well it works. The trustees of a hospital whose major problem is recruiting physicians to practice in a rural area obviously aren't going to spend any time worrying about the real estate acquisition or house staff organization that may be the principal preoccupation of the city hospital board. Thus there can be no prescription for board function that is suitable for everybody, any more than there are any magic numbers or formulas for board size and composition.

Another determination that every institution has to work out for itself is the proper and appropriate division of authority and responsibility between the board of trustees and the administration. Ask anybody having anything to do with hospitals to say what the board does and what the administration does, and the quick answer is going to be, "The board establishes policy, and the administration executes it." Of course, it isn't that easy. In some areas the distinction serves well enough, as when trustees may set forth as policy that all purchases in excess of $500, say, must be made on competitive bids, and all in excess of $5,000 must be approved by the executive committee. No arguments, no problems. But what about turbulent areas like reimbursement, legal action, labor relations, medical practice? Where conditions affecting hospital solvency, liability, or patient care may change from day to day, policies that are necessarily general in nature can provide little guidance. When anesthesiologists walked out of San Francisco hospitals during the malpractice dispute in May 1975 and surgeries were shut down except for life-threatening emergencies, there could be no policies telling management how to cope with the immediate problems of vanishing cash, idle staffs, and agonizing decisions concerning the disposition of patients seeking care. A San Francisco trustee told what it was like: "The hospital began to empty out. Occupancy dropped to 70 percent, 60 percent, 50 percent. Units were closed. Employees were laid off. Hospitals were losing an estimated $200,000 a day and having difficulty meeting their payrolls. One paid employees by stretching the checks out over a three-day period. Another had individual trustees personally guarantee a bank loan. Surgery for a malignancy was not considered life-threatening; we had to turn those patients away. A fractured elbow or hip wasn't life-threatening; the patients were strapped up and moved. Letters and telegrams poured in as the public outcry mounted."[2]

The immediate crisis in San Francisco was resolved when the governor called a special session of the legislature to consider malpractice relief and the doctors went back to work, but trustees of the hospitals there will be coping with the financial, legal, patient care, medical staff, and public relations aftermath for years, and unquestionably some new policies and practices will result. Meanwhile, boards elsewhere can be warned. How well are their policies geared to handle a sudden exodus of doctors and patients? It can be argued, of course, that no policy decision can protect against unexpected disaster. But knowing that such a thing can happen, boards can examine possible ways of preventing the eventuality from occurring and minimizing the impact if it should happen anyway. All hospitals have disaster plans, but not all hospitals have had disasters. Most hospitals have policies determining the position to be taken if a union should start a drive to organize employees, even though many have not yet had to face the situation. Policies governing routine events—admission, discharge, payment, employment, staff appointments, investment, purchasing—evolve over time and can be adjusted with changing circumstance. In these aspects of the hospital's daily activities, moreover, it isn't too difficult to figure out what the trustees should do and what the managers should do. The policies are there; the managers act; the trustees monitor and react. The confusions about board and administrative function arise for the most part out of new and unexpected conditions and out of the complexities of medical staff jurisdiction.

Listen in on any discussion among hospital trustees, and the worries are about the same. Here, for example, are excerpts from a tape recording made in a room where a dozen or so trustees from as many hospitals were visiting with a reporter following one of their regional conferences. What worries you most? the reporter had asked.

"They say you have to do this and you have to do that, and these are government regulations, so you do it even when it doesn't make sense."

"This quality control. We know we have to do it, but the staff thinks it's meddling."

"They think their turf is being invaded."

"We're policemen, really. Policemen keeping the staff and the administration honest."

"It's hard to get knowledgeable about hospitals."

"You've got to plead with them, and then get it half done, but in your own business they wouldn't be there long."

"We know we have the responsibility, but the staff just doesn't believe it."

"How far can we go with this primary care? Who's paying for it?"

"What will the new Medicare reimbursement limits cost us?"

"The doctors say we need tomography now, but the planning agency won't make up their minds."

"If they can't get their malpractice insurance renewed, they say they're going to quit practicing."

"Consumerism is one of the fundamental concerns."

"I think we're aware of a great responsibility to the public."

Awareness of a great responsibility, accompanied by frustration when the means for meeting it keep slipping out of reach because of outside interference and inside independence. This may come as close as anybody can get to fixing the latitude and longitude of hospital trusteeship in the 1970s. To examine the state of the art of overcoming the frustration and discharging the responsibility has been the purpose of this inquiry. What boards of trustees should do has been described many times in position papers, guidelines, manuals, textbooks, and articles, and nearly every hospital has its own manual setting forth the institution's policies and procedures for everything from abortions to autopsies. Everything that has been listed in these prescriptions, and everything trustees work at and worry about, relate in one way or another to these essential functions of the hospital board: (1) ensure survival, (2) set goals, (3) make plans, (4) organize resources, (5) delegate authority, (6) measure performance, and (7) initiate change.

Management does all these things, too, but the distinction between making policy and executing it doesn't always stand up, because (1) the administrator who isn't helping to formulate policy isn't doing his job; (2) the board that stays completely out of operations probably isn't doing its job, either; and (3) policy shades into operations and operations into policy, and there are times when it isn't possible to tell which is which. The way things seem to work in the real world, the difference between what the board does and what the administration does is not so much in policy as it is in scope. Administration's safeguards and goals and plans and resources and authorities and measurements and changes are generally, though not always, *within* those established by the board, and the keys to the success of the relationship, if not the success of the institution, are in the acts of delegation and retention of authority. These require understanding and grace on both sides. Without either quality, the relationship abrades; without both, it fails. It isn't by accident that all the prescriptions and guidelines and position papers say, as they all do, that the most important single responsibility of the hospital board of trustees is the selection and appointment of the chief executive officer. When the right administrator is matched with the right board, differences of function vanish and the acts of retention and delegation are as natural as breathing in and breathing out.

5.　WHO'S IN CHARGE AROUND HERE?

"If you're going to think business, then you'd better get like business," said plainspoken John C. Sturgis, who had been a hospital trustee, or director, as he insists the position should be called, for 25 years but was still a comparatively young man when he quit his bank job a few years ago to become a full-time hospital executive. Mr. Sturgis is impatient with the idea that there is a vast difference between management in the hospital and management in business. "One of the great problems we've had in the hospital is that we tried to view it as something entirely different," he said during an interview in his office at Chicago's Northwestern Memorial Hospital, where one of his first acts was to change the titles. Trustees became directors, and "Would you believe it? The head guy was still superintendent! Everybody knows the superintendent is a guy down in the high school gym. In America, what the guy next door drives, and what his title is, is meaningful. I wanted to put it into language that Americans understand: The boss is president. It's that simple. It's important to get all the titles the same way: vice-president of operations, vice-president of finance. Get away from 'administrator' and all that baloney. Nobody knows what the hell an administrator is and cares less."

Mr. Sturgis is not unmindful of the special problems of management and control created by the offstage voice of the medical staff. "We have this one difference that anybody running a business would find queer," he acknowledged, "but it's the only one, and I don't like to emphasize it because then it gets used as an excuse for running this business differently. But it is true that if the chief of staff walks in here one morning and tells me to stuff it in my ear, I'll put up with quite a bit of it, because I recognize that this is one odd element of our management. In a bank you would probably unload him, you know, or you wouldn't put up with much of it."

According to Mr. Sturgis, who is now chairman of the executive committee of Northwestern Memorial, which was created by the merger of the former Passavant Memorial Hospital and Chicago Wesley Memorial Hospital, of which he was a director and president, there are two things to remember about doctors: "The first thing is, we never teach them any business; that's not their fault, it's ours. The second thing is that the doctor is a small god from the time he is about 22 years old. He has never been anybody's right-hand man. He's never been squashed as a little credit clerk in the back of the bank or the corporation. He's never worked under the lash of many managers as he grows up and matures to become an executive who can look back with some understanding and some sympathy for the people below him. He's been deified by the public almost from day one, and never really reported to anyone." That's not how anybody but Jack Sturgis would describe a career that included an internship, perhaps, but he isn't impressed. "The tough old chief who hammered them all to death was mostly in old movies and is actually a rarity today."

For all his tough talk, Jack Sturgis has great respect and admiration for physicians. "No one will ever build a statue to a hospital executive," he said. "To doctors and nurses, yes, and properly so, because their talents are what we sell." But he doesn't think directors should be intimidated by them. He considers open communication among board, administration, and staff essential to effective management. When he first came to Wesley, he said, "I told the doctors, 'You're going to put me on your boards, and I'm going to put you on ours. You're going to be on our committees, and I'm going to sit on yours, with other directors as needed. This business of not talking to each other is going to end.' " That doesn't solve all the problems, he conceded. "The chiefs and I have fought like hell at various times. We've Indian-wrestled in the halls, and yet it has worked out all right. Too often in the past, doctors had appealed to their favorite board members to push some program in opposition to the chief executive officer. I've had just one call in six years from a director who interceded for a doctor. If your door is always open, you have a right to insist that the medical staff take up their problems with you and not the directors."

Indian wrestling with doctors and avoidance of cocktail party conferences of doctors and directors are not among the listed skills directors commonly seek in recruiting an executive, but the successful executive of any enterprise is usually an artful negotiator who knows when to stand fast, when to give ground, and when to charge. Nowhere else is the blend of character, intelligence, and sensitivity that produces this quality more important to effective management than it is in the hospital, where the executive must deal with physicians who stand outside the administrative hierarchy but whose decisions and actions have everything to do with the success of the institution. When Peter Drucker, the management consultant who is everybody's favorite guru of executives, described the hospital as the most complex and sophisticated organization in the world, it is unlikely that he was thinking about the chart of accounts or the linen supply system. As a less celebrated observer said, "Every industry has its problems, but nobody else has doctors."

From the standpoint of trustees or directors, another difficulty is that the methods of measuring management performance include consideration of values that for most businessmen are arcane, if not completely unfathomable. Given a reasonable regard for the protection of assets over time, the bottom line is a generally faithful guide to the quality of management performance in industry. Certainly the bottom line is not to be disregarded altogether in the hospital, but neither can it be accepted as infallible; an apparently comfortable margin may have been achieved at the expense of adequate staffing on the nursing floors, for example, or an alarming shortfall in needed cash may develop because a public agency whose patients can't be turned away is months behind in its payments for their services. The management of the San Francisco hospitals that were drained of surgical patients when the anesthesiologists debouched in the malpractice retreat may have performed near miracles to keep the hospitals open, but only the empty beds were reflected in the bottom line.

This is not to say that trustees have no indexes by which to judge how well their managers are performing or to answer the question they like to ask administrators, "How are we doing?" Far from it. There are all kinds of standards. Performance compared to budgets that have been examined and approved by the board is a reliable guide, for openers. Others that follow quickly are: costs per patient day and costs per case by departments, which can be compared to those of other institutions of like size and services; cash on hand, payables, and receivables in relation to revenue; ratios of payroll to total expense, staffing to numbers of patients, work performed or output to employee man-hours.

These and other financial and statistical yardsticks are as familiar to hospital administrators, and to some trustees, or super trustees, as yards gained and tackles made are to the football coach. But these don't tell the whole complex story of hospital management performance, either, by any means. Instead, they must be viewed in the light cast by a whole array of other indexes: admissions, discharges, outpatient visits, births, deaths, operations, occupancy, length of stay, tests and procedures performed, services rendered, medications given—many of these by department, or by diagnosis, or both.

Some standards based on these data have been known and used for years, others have been developed just recently, and some are still emerging. All these—there are now statistical norms in general use for upward of 400 diagnoses—are tricky guides, but the only ones there are, to the quality of the medical care being rendered in the institution, once considered the doctors' business and out of bounds for trustees and administrators but now held by courts, accreditation authorities, and paying agencies to be, to some degree and under some circumstances, the responsibility of the hospital and therefore of its management and governing board. The trustee or administrator may never be able to recite the indications for cholesystectomy, but he had better know if one of his surgeons has been operating in the absence of those considered to be the acceptable minimum. Financial and statistical data, standards, and norms by size and type of hospital, by region, and by other appropriate breakdowns may be furnished to hospitals in reports from Hospital Administrative Services, a service offered by the American Hospital Association. Medical data in similar detail are available from the Commission on Professional and Hospital Activities, an agency sponsored by the AHA, American College of Surgeons, American College of Physicians, and Southwestern Michigan Hospital Council.

Finally, there is a whole other spectrum of answers to the question "How are we doing?" for which there are no ratios or indexes or standards at all, and none in sight. These are all the values that come under the rubric "care," as opposed to "cure." There are some who think that care is less important now than it was years ago when kindness, sympathy, and encouragement were a larger part of all that doctors and nurses could do for their patients. But there are others—and more of them all the time—who think care in this sense is an important element of hospital service that has been neglected in the era of technology and specialization and now needs to be restored and reemphasized. "People who are troubled, who are in pain, who are disabled, want to see someone, to talk to someone, to share their troubles with someone," says the health economist Victor R. Fuchs. "As much as a cure, they want sympathy, reassurance, encouragement. They want explanations: 'Why did this happen?' 'How long will it last?' They want justifications: 'Should I stay home from work?' 'Should I have any more children?' Above all, they want someone who *cares*."[1]

What can trustees and administrators do about the "care" component of hospital service? Social and behavioral scientists who have analyzed hospitals are convinced that caring, like efficiency, has to come from the top and is basically a product of how hospital employees at all levels feel about their jobs, and thus it is something that management, as well as physicians and nurses, are responsible for. Feelings are not susceptible of precise measurement, perhaps, but they can be gauged to some extent by attitude surveys and other methods known to personnel experts. Jack Sturgis has relied on an instrument he describes as the "bitching level." Bitching is inevitable in any organization, he believes. "There's a certain decibel level of bitching every day, and I don't want to be held accountable for that." But watch out for peaks in the bitching chart. "I'll be accountable for the rises when they should be listened to," he said. "If you ever stop and listen in an elevator, they're always talking about their boss, or what's wrong in the department, or how Harry is doing. Some level of this is necessary and acceptable. No problem." For trustees and administrators who don't trust their elevator ears, there are more formal and expensive, if not any more reliable, means of assessing the emotional atmosphere of the hospital and finding another part of the answer to "How are we doing?"

Because the board-staff-administration complex is such an intricate web of relationships combining cognate interests and disparate backgrounds and responsibilities, there are times when all the indicators and answers are favorable but something is still obviously wrong. A trustee of a hospital that had changed administrators just a few years ago when management of finances got out of hand told this story of continued tribulation:

"We brought consultants in and spent $60,000 to come up with the same answers we could have got from our own auditors, and we got a nice written report saying in effect, "Get a new manager and let him manage." So we went out and got new management that wouldn't have taken the job without this background, so in a sense the report was worthwhile. Almost immediately, the financial side of the institution was changed. We got into the black and have been in the black ever since, and from the financial point of view everything is working beautifully.

"On the other hand, the new management is creating all kinds of problems with some of the older people on the board, because they feel they cannot go down and talk to the people at the hospital, as they always used to do in the old days. Or, they can talk to them all they want so long as they don't tell them what to do, but if they start telling them what to do, we have problems. Yet some of the trustees felt that they aren't being productive on the board if they can't tell people what to do in the hospital, which is, of course, a misunderstanding of the function and responsibility of a trustee for general direction, depending on the organization to accomplish what the board sets as its objectives. I tried for a while to get them to adopt the corporate form of organization, thinking it would help to clarify the relationship, but the president of the board thought it would be a demotion if he became chairman, so I dropped it.

"Some people on the board still feel they have to go back and get involved in every decision at the hospital. Policymaking doesn't answer it for them, but the administration side feels very strongly that it should be told what the policy is and allowed to function within that. So there are conflicts. Childish things, such as the president is now objecting strongly because the administrator is signing letters of thanks to the people who make contributions to the hospital. He thinks it's degrading, because the president ought to be signing the letters. Well I think he should be, too, but for a different reason altogether: He and the board members have the substantial contacts in the community that should be played up and strengthened, and letters from the president would help more than letters from the administrator do. The administrator doesn't want people from the board going down to the hospital telling department heads what to do, and I agree with that completely. On the other hand, he's left the impression, at least with some of these people, that he doesn't want them in the hospital at all, and they think it's because he's afraid they will find out something and use it against him. It's a constant battle.

"One of the fringe benefits in the administrator's contract is that he is allowed to go to four or five meetings a year, which I think is perfectly in order. But every once in a while he wants to go to another one when some board members think he should stay at the hospital, so we have more battles. All kinds of little things like this have gone on, and it just drives you crazy, because it interferes with what we are trying to accomplish here. It doesn't have to happen that way at all, and we've just gone around and around on it.

"On the medical side, the doctors used to go directly to board members, than a board member would beg for them for something, and this interferes with proper management. So finally we put the medical director and the president of the staff on the board, and they serve on all the committees, and then when these problems with board members came up at the meetings, several people wanted to ask the medical director and administrator to leave, even though they were members of the board with the right to vote. I objected strenuously to that. If we can't talk it out in the open, with them there, why it's all wrong. If they're board members, they have as much right to be there as anybody else has, and they ought to have the right to defend themselves. We finally voted on it, and it was voted that they should stay.

"I think that in the end this may have stopped some of the criticism of the administration. Some of the cases that were brought up involved conflicts of interest of some of the people on the board who were complaining. As a result of that, a committee on governance was appointed to look into these cases and the criticisms of management generally, and every member of the board who wanted to was invited to come and testify. Out of some 27 or 28 board members, about five or six had something to say. The things they had to say were very minor, fundamentally. Maybe the administration wasn't considerate enough of their interests and dedication to the hospital. That's a reasonable view, but they really didn't have much; there was no substance to it at all. In fact, they all admit that the management of the institution has been great. Maybe the personalities weren't as nice as they should be. That's really where we came out."

The fact that the episodes related by this trustee seem insubstantial, as he has described them, does not necessarily mean that they are therefore inconsequential. Any action or circumstance that results in continuing conflict, a "constant battle," has to be taken seriously, because it is draining away attention and energy that ought to be directed instead toward the purposes of the enterprise. So, in spite of the administrator's recognized managerial competence, and in spite of the fact that his position or the principle he considered to be at stake in the continuing dispute was unquestionably right, to the extent that there can be right and wrong in such matters, this has to be put down as a failure of management. It was a less serious failure than that of the predecessor who lost control of finances, to be sure, but a failure nevertheless. The trustee called it a matter of personality, and the administrator saw it as a matter of defending his authority against improper encroachment, and they may both have been right. But the point is that there was probably a way for the board members' need to feel important to be satisfied without any substantive surrender of the administrator's authority, and if such a way isn't discovered in time, the relationship will fail. If this should happen, the administrator may have won the battle, but he will have lost the war.

All the textbooks, manuals, and articles that have been written for hospital trustees emphasize that the trustees must let the managers manage without interfering in the day-to-day operations of the institution. Administrators are trained to believe this is the way it should happen, but only intuition or experience can tell them what to do when it doesn't. There are circumstances, of course, where interference cannot be tolerated, but the one described here doesn't appear to have been one of them. Like Indian wrestling, the fine art of treating molehills as molehills is an unlisted skill that can be learned but not taught. It is probably as important to the success of the board-administration relationship as any other desirable quality sought for by a hospital board recruiting an administrator, and a lot harder to identify in a candidate during an interview. The closest any job specification ever comes to defining it is in the line reading "must get along well with people," or some such, and no board or search committee ever interviewed a candidate who didn't, either on the record or in the interview, get along with people. The committee that is willing to probe the record, and not all of them are, may find clues beneath a resignation that is explained away as a "clash of personalities," and the committee that is unusually perceptive may conclude that the candidate who has always been right is probably wrong. The job specifications can be copied out of any textbook and matched against the visible record, but there are absolutely no easy ways to determine in advance how well any candidate is going to wear under the hammering multipressures of hospital management.

Of course, the specifications can't literally be copied out of any textbook but need to be tailored to the institution's perceived needs for expertise and experience in, say, finance, or medical staff organization, or planning. As the job of administrator or president or chief executive officer has become more and more exacting in recent years, hospitals have increasingly turned to management consultants or executive search firms, most of which have some experience, at least, in recruiting executives for hospital administration responsibilities. Usually, the experienced executive searcher, following interviews with the board members involved, will find some gaps in the specifications prepared by the board and spend some time revising these.

"The firm did a survey of the hospital and its needs as these were seen from both the management and board points of view," a trustee told an acquaintance recently, describing a search that was still going on at the time. "The ideal candidate will walk on water. I damn near died when I read the qualities a chief executive of a hospital like this should have. It is an immense bill of goods, partly just to run the business, and partly to get along with and contribute to the effectiveness of the medical staff, and the need to be familiar with what is going on in the field politically, legislatively, and professionally. It's a hell of a job, and I don't think any man is ever going to come along who is equally strong in all these features. So what we are trying to do is to find someone who is particularly outstanding in one or more of them, and then fill in underneath him as we may need to, either from the inside or the outside. Once we find out who he is, we can determine what assistance he may need."

This was a teaching hospital, and the trustee was asked whether the board committee or the head-hunter thought the executive should be a physician. "I would say we have a fairly open mind," he replied. "He could be a physician, but if he isn't, we're thinking about creating a specific medical position in the management group. From my own experience, however, I would say there have been both successes and failures among both medical and nonmedical executives in this kind of job. What we're looking at are the individual's basic qualifications and history, and we're not worrying too much about whether or not he has an MD." The search firm had first narrowed the field down to about 60 candidates, the trustee reported, then picked 30 of these for a second look. From these it would select the ones to be interviewed, and, finally, choose not more than three or four for interviews with the board's own search committee. The process would take six to nine months from beginning to end. "It's a tough job," he concluded. "But I've got a lot of confidence in the people on that committee. They're pretty good."

In his report to the New York hospitals, Russell Nelson, M.D., addressed the notion that the chief executive officer of a teaching hospital had to be a physician because "only a physician can understand physicians' problems and attitudes," as it has so often been stated. Experience in the health institutional field is an absolute requirement for successful executive performance, he acknowledged, but "it is certainly not true that only a physician can understand these relationships and respond appropriately. Nor is it true that physicians on the staffs will accept direction only from another physician. In addition to the required experience, the requisite qualities include knowledge of organizational principles and modern management practice, the ability to comprehend and articulate the goals and missions of the enterprise, the character to stand up to pressure and make fair judgments, the capacity to motivate and lead others toward common goals, and, finally, a quality which has been described as a sense of fitness or balance."[2]

Dr. Nelson quoted a colleague on the last-named quality: "Being an administrator is more of a strain on the character than on the intellect. The people around you often make life uncomfortable and tax your endurance. The mark of an administrator is often his ability to tolerate an ambiguous situation. If the frustration tolerance is low, the administrator will not be effective." The administrator Dr. Nelson was quoting in his report was John H. Knowles, M.D., who was general director of the Massachusetts General Hospital for 10 years and then became president of the Rockefeller Foundation, and it is possible, at least, that his "tolerance of ambiguity" would include a fair measure of Indian wrestling and treating molehills as molehills.

Neither of these skills is to be found in the list of chief executive officer's responsibilities included in the American Hospital Association's Management

Review Program, but it is doubtful that the duties that are included could all be performed satisfactorily without, at very least, a sense of balance. They are:
1. Submitting for approval a plan of organization for the conduct of hospital operation and recommending changes when necessary.
2. Preparing a plan for the achievement of the hospital's specific objectives and periodically reviewing and evaluating it.
3. Selecting, employing, controlling, and discharging all employees.
4. Submitting for approval an annual budget showing expected receipts and expenditures.
5. Recommending the rates to be charged for hospital services.
6. Having charge and custody of and being responsible for all operating funds of the corporation.
7. Maintaining all physical properties in a good state of repair and operating condition.
8. Representing the hospital in its relationships with other health agencies.
9. Serving as liaison and channel of communications between the governing board or its committees and the medical staff.
10. Assisting the medical staff with its organizational and medical-administrative problems and responsibilities.
11. Submitting to the governing board reports showing the professional service and financial experience of the hospital, and submitting such special reports as may be requested by the governing board.
12. Advising the governing board on matters of policy formulation.

In addition, the AHA says in a postscript to this catalog of responsibilities, the chief executive or his delegate is expected to attend all meetings of the governing board and its committees, and to advise and keep "the governing board currently informed on significant trends which enable it to carry out its function of policy formulation . . . [including] information [on] and explanation of (1) significant economic, legislative, and social factors which influence the hospital field in general and this hospital in particular; (2) activities of local, state, and national organizations which are related to the hospital's program of service; (3) conditions within the hospital which may require action by the governing board; [and] (4) technical and scientific advances in the health field."[3]

Considering this formidable configuration of function, it is possible to conclude as Dr. Nelson did that "the task of the hospital executive today may be described as a management exercise requiring an abundant fund of knowledge and an extraordinary variety of skills, chief among which is that of negotiation. Like the master of simultaneous chess who moves from table to table making instant transitions of adversaries, situations, strategies, decisions, and actions, the hospital executive moves through his succession of negotiations with patients, families, employees, physicians, trustees, community groups, insurers, bankers, planners, government officials, politicians, and reporters, making arrangements and accommodations in the interests of the institution, and the people and community and mission the institution serves. It is always possible for an adversary, or an interested party, or an observer of any segment of any of the negotiations to find fault with the executive's assessment of the situation, or his strategy, or a decision that is made, or an action that is taken, but the entire performance has to be measured in the context of the full circle of negotiations. Thus whoever is constrained to make a judgment would do well to remember that no matter where he sits in the circle, there is somebody on the other side."[4]

It is a thought for trustees.

Successful businessmen who become hospital trustees have been known to exhibit lapses of judgment in their hospital decisions that they would be the first to denounce in their offices downtown. As one critic has said, "When they come to a hospital board meeting, they seem to have left their business brains in the pocket of another suit."

Why does it happen? When such lapses occur, more often than not it is in connection with a matter of medical affairs. Thus the chairman of the board of a giant corporation who was also board chairman of a large hospital not long ago sought to solve a troublesome but essentially minor problem of medical organization by hiring a full-time medical executive and putting him in charge of the hospital's medical faculty and staff, outside the jurisdiction of the incumbent executive vice-president, whose performance was generally regarded as outstanding. In one stroke, the chairman created an impossible two-headed monster that any business school undergraduate would have told him couldn't possibly work, muddied the channels of communication and authority beyond all comprehension, worsened instead of solving the problems of medical organization, and within a few months caused the respected executive vice-president to flee into early retirement. Any executive making a similar move in the complex of companies headed by the chairman would have been fired out of hand.

Invariably, trustees who are asked how such things can happen at first deny that they themselves could be guilty of any such aberrant behavior. Then, on reflection, they may admit that they are uncomfortable and sometimes thrown off stride by the presence of decision makers who are in the organization but somehow immune to the chain of command. "I put up with a lot of things up there," a corporate executive said, referring to the hospital he serves as a board member, "that I wouldn't stand for around here"—meaning corporate headquarters on Park Avenue. Asked what kind of things he had in mind, he thought a minute and said, "Well, for example, we'll have a board or committee meeting and decide something should be done right away, with the administrator and medical director or chief of staff sitting there agreeing with everything that's being said. Then a month goes by, or maybe it's three months, and you find out absolutely nothing has happened. Nothing!" He glared at the interviewer. "You can bet your ear that couldn't happen down here! But when you ask for an explanation, it turns out to be something like 'the doctors didn't seem to be ready for it.' So instead of blowing the lid off, you back away." At the expense of elevated trustee blood pressure in some cases, obviously.

It isn't *always* medical affairs that are involved; sometimes trustees who know better are guilty of faulty judgment in hospital decisions that are purely managerial. Thus a common flaw found in hospital organizations by business analysts and management consultants experienced in hospital assignments is lack of strength in depth in the executive structure. Trustees whose banks or factories are abundantly staffed with vice-presidents of everything from air conditioning to washrooms have sometimes appeared to think that a $20 million a year hospital business can be run by a single administrator with a couple of low-salaried, anonymous assistants. It doesn't make sense.

Fortunately, trustees are learning that it can't be done that way anymore, given the constantly swelling list of burdensome executive responsibilities, and hospitals are being staffed with qualified specialists in all the principal phases of operations, leaving chief executives freer than they have been in the past to focus their attention on the changing political, social, and professional environments in which the hospital operates and on the vital functions of planning and public relations. The medical director of a hospital that has chronically lacked an adequate staff of executives with needed special knowledge and skills was a sympathetic observer of the problems plaguing the capable but overworked administrator. "We're simply treading water," he said. "The harassment of administrators under today's conditions is such that they don't have time for an orderly approach to problems. They respond to crises instead of developing the things that are needed for the future. The trustees have a planning committee, and so does the medical board, but these are not adequate substitutes for one full-time person giving real thought to plans for the future. The right kind of administrative leadership would permit creative thinking."

Lack of depth in management is responsible for another recurring problem in the hospital field: the need always to look outside when the time comes to seek a replacement at the top, with all the inevitable losses of time and control that follow while the new chief executive is learning his way around and treading cautiously. A hospital with a dozen qualified vice-presidents or division heads can test and observe these younger executives on the job, then make a selection from among known performers and prepare for orderly succession when it becomes necessary, as most large corporations have been doing for years. The outside appointee, with all his built-in handicaps, is the rule among hospital executives but the exception in business.

Here is what the head of a huge merchandising empire had to say about the way top executives are developed in his business: "First, promising young executives are chosen for our training program, and following this they are given merchandising management responsibilities at branch stores with increasingly large sales, payrolls, and problems. Then a few of them are brought in here to the corporate offices, where they get a succession of assignments. They learn by doing, in other words, until they are ready for major executive responsibility." Ironically, but not uncharacteristically, this man also had been chairman of the board of trustees of a large hospital whose administrator was getting along as well as he could with a financial vice-president, an all-purpose assistant, and a part-time medical director. "The hospital is a big business," the trustee had said in the course of the conversation about executive development, "and the same principles of management have to be followed." They could be, but it doesn't always happen.

"Health administration is planning, organizing, directing, controlling, coordinating, and evaluating the resources and procedures by which needs and demands for health and medical care and a healthful environment are fulfilled, by the provision of specific services to individual clients, organizations, and communities," said the report of a Commission on Education for Health Administration in 1974. "Responsibilities and functions involved in this process vary from one health or medical care organization to another, from one level of activity to another, and from one time to another. The Commission strongly encourages those with responsibility for carrying out the health administration process to assume a leadership role. For this role to be fulfilled, health administrators must acquire and demonstrate competence that ranks them as peers of the providers of direct services and enables them to be supported by others in the system, by government, and by the public; administrative concern for fiscal matters and efficient use of resources must be balanced by concern for promotion and maintenance of health, equitable access to and high quality of services, and public accountability in all aspects of administrative performance; there must be impetus and strong support from policymakers and the public for achieving balance between pressures for fiscal accountability and accountabilities for the character and quality of the services provided; and relationships between health administration and other human services administration in welfare agencies, legal agencies and primary and secondary education must be recognized and strengthened."[5]

In other words, there's a lot to be done.

6. ALL THE CARE FOR ALL THE PATIENTS ALL THE TIME

"Thou'dst shun a bear, but if thy flight lay toward the roaring sea thou'dst meet the bear in the mouth," said King Lear, "for where the greater malady is fixed, the lesser is scarce felt." Hospital trustees who consider that the greater malady today is the necessity for maintaining medical standards and avoiding the kind of liability that devolved on the hospitals in the *Darling*[1] and *Nork*[2] cases are less inclined to be uptight about the money problems besetting their hospitals under restrictive reimbursement policies.

One who thinks medical liability is the lesser malady is a trustee of a New York hospital whose outpatient clinics and emergency departments are bursting with neighborhood patients demanding services nobody is willing to pay for at anything like what they cost. "We just can't go on the way we are," he said. "If we can't get the payments increased, we're going to have to start closing the doors." Under these circumstances the board doesn't worry much about medical problems, he said, adding that he didn't think it would make much sense to have physicians as trustees. "The things we talk about at board and executive committee meetings are not the doctors' business anyway. The medical staff is like a club. The referrals and problems stay inside the club, and I don't think we would want to change this, even if we thought we could."

Trustees elsewhere view medical liability as the roaring sea and worry more about utilization review, quality assurance, and the rising number of states in which recent court decisions have either stated outright or are being interpreted as having said that the governing board and administration have not done their full duty to their patients when they have simply made certain the mechanisms for quality assessment are in place and left it up to the doctors to make them work.

But whether it is medicine or money that predominates in the discussions at board meetings, the fact is that boards of trustees today don't get to choose between the greater and lesser maladies. They have to meet them both in the mouth at the same time, and the two are not unrelated, because it is the paying agencies, and chiefly the federal government, that are insisting on effective utilization review to cut down payments for services that can't be demonstrated to be medically necessary; effective utilization review costs money, and it isn't entirely clear yet who is going to pay for it, and how much.

Hospital responsibility for the quality of medical care is not what anybody could call a new concept. More than 60 years ago a Boston surgeon, E. A. Codman, M.D., had instituted a system of outcomes measurement in the department of surgery at the Massachusetts General Hospital and was agitating among his colleagues in the Massachusetts Medical Society and among the trustees of the hospital for the wide-scale adoption of his scheme, which he insisted was a safeguard the hospital owed its patients. In part because the concept *was* in fact a radical one for that time, and in part because Dr. Codman's methods of publicizing his views were not always in keeping with what was considered to be proper medical decorum, he was ostracized, socially and professionally, for his pains. However, he persisted in the pursuit of his objectives and later became one of the founding members of the American College of Surgeons and chairman of its first committee on hospital standardization.

Owing in large part to the dedicated efforts of Malcolm T. MacEachern, M.D., who directed the ACS hospital standardization program for more than 30 years, it became the recognized means of identifying hospitals that observed what were considered to be the acceptable standards for those years, including governing boards and organized medical staffs that were assumed to be self-governing, at least to the extent of having known requirements for staff appointments and privileges and censuring transgressors. Moreover, with increasing specialization of medical practice, the standards for approval in the program were elevated over the years, though the methods for enforcing them never advanced much beyond the finger-pointing stage.

Commenting not long ago on the introduction of a new standard on the quality of professional services by the Joint Commission on Accreditation of Hospitals, which had taken over the American College of Surgeons program in 1951 and has been the chief vehicle for certifying hospital excellence since that time, John D. Porterfield, M.D., director of the commission, remarked that the health industry "periodically scratches irritably at the itching of JCAH, its conscience, objecting to its incursive demands, but nevertheless cherishing its continuation. The consumers and their sometime voice, the government, deride it as the fox in the chicken coop, the whitewash squad, and other appellations less printable, yet depend on it in many ways as at least the best game in town."[3] Always with the quality of patient care as its primary objective, the JCAH for years had concentrated on the environment of health care services and on measurable input criteria, such as the educational qualifications of physicians and other hospital personnel, Dr. Porterfield explained, and this had been necessary because of the limitations of the evaluation process and the need to evaluate measurable dimensions. Even so, he said, "JCAH continued to urge attention to concurrent and reflective appraisal of the quality of services, with a view to improvement in practice."*

Over the past few years, however, new methods have been developed for the objective, efficient evaluation of the quality of care. "With the mounting frustrations of a more sophisticated and skeptical consumer public, there can be no unnecessary delay in the application of these techniques," Dr. Porterfield declared. Hence the new standard: "The hospital shall demonstrate that the quality of care provided to all patients is consistently optimal by continuously evaluating it through reliable and valid measures. Where the quality of care is shown to be less than optimal, improvement in quality shall be demonstrated." The demonstration of quality is accomplished by measurement of actual care against specific criteria established or adapted by the medical staff, it is explained. Whatever their source, the criteria include expected patient outcomes, such as health status at discharge, complications, and other appropriate data, and, when observed outcomes fall short of expectations, criteria reflecting desirable processes of care are to be applied. Criteria also include validation of the diagnosis and justification for admission and for surgery and whatever other procedures and services may be employed.

----

*Over the years, physicians from time to time have protested JCAH demands on their time and attention to medical records, staff meetings and conferences, and other evidence that controls on quality are in place, objecting that these measures in effect were means of policing the medical profession— a term JCAH abhors. Thus the JCAH and the AHA were horrified some years ago when science writer Don Robinson in a magazine article referred to Dr. Porterfield's predecessor, Kenneth Babcock, M.D., as a medical policeman. Robinson was unmoved. "He looks like a policeman, he talks like a policeman, he acts like a policeman, and as far as I am concerned, he *is* a policeman," Robinson told an AHA representative.[4]

"Variations from the established criteria shall be identified and justified," the JCAH said in an interpretation of the standard. "In actual practice, variations from criteria are often fully justified, but evidence for such justification must appear in the patient medical record, and the reason for justification must be explicitly stated by the professionals evaluating care." Justifications that are not judged to be satisfactory by the staff committee or group responsible for evaluating care must then be analyzed, and, "if analysis indicates inappropriate patterns of patient care, action must be taken to correct problems. Such action should be specific to the problem and may include educational or training programs, amended policies or procedures, increased or realigned staffing, provision of new equipment or facilities, or adjustments in staff privileges," the JCAH said. "The entire patient care evaluation activity must be documented and its results reported. The general findings of and specific recommendations from evaluation studies conducted by the medical staff must be reported to the executive committee of the staff, the chief of staff, the chief executive officer of the hospital, and the governing body." The commission also expects that the results of medical care evaluation will be carried over into other medical staff functions such as reappointments to staff membership and privileges, controls of utilization of beds and other facilities and services, continued monitoring of practice, and provision of educational opportunities for staff members.

Beginning in 1975, the JCAH started to examine and evaluate the medical audit and evaluation systems in use in hospitals against these essentials. It is compliance with the fundamental principles of medical care evaluation, and not the specific system in use, that is examined. "With the availability of a variety of feasible techniques, JCAH has been able to apply the same evaluative approach to direct-services quality assurance programs that it has continually done in the area of environmental impact on quality," Dr. Porterfield said.

There is no lack of systems for the hospital seeking guidance to choose from. The JCAH itself has published a Performance Evaluation Procedure for Auditing and Evaluating Patient Care (PEP) and conducts educational workshops for hospital personnel with step-by-step instruction in the initiation and conduct of the procedure. The American Hospital Association's Quality Assurance Program for Medical Care in the Hospital (QAP) contains a series of guidelines for implementing programs of admissions review, continued stay review, discharge planning, and medical care evaluation that can be adapted for individual hospital use to demonstrate that resources are being used efficiently and that patient care performance quality standards are being met. The AHA has also been conducting training sessions for hospital personnel, with emphasis on the training of non-physician utilization review coordinators whose basic function is to examine performance data against criteria, so that physician time will be used only in consideration of variations whose justification requires professional judgment. Reporting the results of a 1973 survey, the AHA said that more than 1,000 hospitals were committed to the implementation of quality assurance as described in the QAP guidelines.

Still another program has been introduced by the Commission on Professional and Hospital Activities (see chapter 5). Called the Quality Assurance Monitor (QAM), this system is designed to provide a practical method for monitoring the quality of care of all patients in the hospital, at the same time furnishing data that permit comparisons with norms of care in other hospitals for the same diagnoses. The QAM manual presents an alphabetical list of the diagnoses that account for 90 percent of all discharges from more than 2,100 hospitals reporting to CPHA from throughout the United States and Canada.

The Blue Cross Association also has a Plan Utilization Review (PUR) program of assistance for Blue Cross Plans wishing to provide their member hospitals with systems for screening claims and conducting utilization review; state and regional systems have been developed by groups in Pennsylvania, Ohio, California, and elsewhere; and many hospitals have developed or are developing their own quality assurance systems, using their own data.

While it has always been possible for a hospital, or, as in the case of Dr. Codman at the Massachusetts General Hospital 60 years ago, a clinical department of a hospital, to establish standards by which the processes and outcomes of patient care could be judged, the standards in the past have generally been crude, and the procedure for applying them in the measurement of care for any large number of patients required more time than anybody with anything else to do could possibly provide. The breakthrough referred to by Dr. Porterfield that has made possible the more precise measurements and their application to large numbers of patients with relative ease has, of course, been the development of computer technology and its use in medical information systems that can assemble, classify, analyze, and display masses of patient data, making it possible, as Vergil N. Slee, M.D., president of the Commission on Professional and Hospital Activities, likes to say, for any hospital to measure the quality of "all the care for all the patients all the time."[5]

Actually, it was the confluence of the emerging technology and the rising demand for more accurate appraisals of care that resulted in the burgeoning interest in quality assurance of the early 1970s, and unquestionably the demand has been occasioned as much by concern for efficient use of resources as by any widespread belief that the care itself was less than satisfactory. It seems likely that the concern of the Congress in approving the Professional Standards Review Organization provisions of the Social Security Amendments of 1972 was chiefly to establish some method of eliminating payment for any unnecessary services in Medicare and Medicaid, whose costs have kept on mounting at an alarming rate ever since they were introduced in 1966, but the protracted argument about whether PSRO was aimed at controlling cost or quality was mostly pointless, since it would obviously have an impact on both, and, as hospital administrators and board members have come to understand, the two are inseparable anyway. An unnecessary admission or overlong stay or unneeded medication or operation subtracts something from quality as surely, if not as obtrusively, as it adds something to cost.

During the long debate on the PSRO program, members of Congress insisted that they were interested not just in cutting down Medicare and Medicaid costs but also in making certain that "the American people are getting full value for the dollars they are paying for health care"—an assurance that seems likely to remain an elusive goal even if PSRO accomplishes everything that was envisioned by its sponsors. "The ultimately perfect vehicle for valid accreditation may never be reached," Dr. Porterfield said when he announced the new JCAH standard for quality of professional services. "The substantial progress of recent years will not dull the continuing search for better methodologies to protect and reinforce the quality of the care of the patient in the most feasible and professionally rational way. This professionally oriented approach to patients' concerns is one advantage of the voluntary system." In a pluralistic system, however, there is always room for other approaches and other goals. Caspar Weinberger, former Secretary of Health, Education, and Welfare, who was not widely beloved among hospital people but was respected by many for his straightforward manner, had said in 1974 that "the cost of health care remains the single most important problem in the industry today, far more serious than the related issues of quality and access."

The PSRO program, which like the rhinoceros has a long gestation period and an odd shape, has developed haltingly since the law was passed in 1972, troubled by many uncertainties of objectives, methods, and funding. The physician groups, set apart from both their medical societies and their hospital staffs, may yet emerge to help achieve the goals envisioned by both Dr. Porterfield and Mr. Weinberger, or they may not accomplish much in either direction and simply add another layer of organization, paper, and expense to an already overburdened system.

Dismissing PSROs in a book called *Medical Nemesis,* published in England in 1974, the priest-educator-social critic Ivan Illich said "the United States is the only country in the world that has launched a national legislative program to assure the quality of care offered in the free market and has left it entirely up to the medical profession to determine what quality is."[6] At the same time, he said that the socialist nations had assumed all the financing of health care but "leave it to the medical profession to define what is needed, how it is done, who may do it, what it should cost, and who should get it." Since the socialist nations also employ the doctors and decide how much they are paid, however, U.S. doctors still appear to have the best deal there is anywhere, and many of them consider that PSROs may offer them the best opportunity to keep the deal.

In late 1975, at any rate, PSROs were in the planning stage or operating under conditional approval from the Department of HEW in more than half the nation's 203 designated PSRO areas. Hospitals had to decide whether to let their area PSROs assume the utilization review (UR) function or seek delegated authority from the PSROs to develop their own systems and do it themselves. Those that already had effective utilization review either had or were requesting delegated authority, and tipping the balance toward hospital-based UR for those still undecided was an emerging policy under which it appeared that Medicare and Medicaid reimbursement would include hospital UR costs. A counterargument being heard in mid-1975 was that physicians relinquishing responsibility for monitoring patient care to PSROs might deflect some of their liability for malpractice in the same direction, if plaintiffs should come to consider that PSROs were responsible for maintaining standards.

Also in 1975, another arm of HEW, the Social Security Administration's Bureau of Health Insurance, had sought to impose new utilization review procedures for Medicare patients, including a requirement that every hospital admission must be reviewed and certified as medically necessary within one working day following the admission, a provision that was considered by hospitals to be unworkable. The AHA protested vigorously on behalf of its member institutions and succeeded in getting the effective date of the new regulations postponed twice. Meanwhile, the American Medical Association had sued the Secretary of HEW, contending that he had exceeded his authority in seeking to impose the regulations and that the one-working-day requirement would unlawfully interfere with the physician's right to practice medicine in accordance with his own professional judgment. A federal judge in Chicago agreed to the extent of granting a temporary injunction restraining the Secretary from enforcing the one-day provision, which was later withdrawn for modification. But it was also clear that the federal government, now paying $24 billion a year for Medicare and Medicaid, and the greater part of that for hospital care, was going to insist on the kind of utilization review that would impose stricter requirements for demonstrating the medical need for hospitalization than have prevailed in the past and that the PSRO program would be the federal monitoring instrument.

Whether it is PSROs, the Social Security Administration, or some other agency that is looking on, however, the thing that is going to make quality assurance work, in the opinion of most of those who have either made it work or seen it work in hospitals, is locally developed criteria. "It's as simple as that," said Clement Brown, M.D., who, as AHA's former director of medical relations, explained how QAP works. "Distantly developed criteria can't do the job, and locally developed criteria can do it." This view was reinforced by Warren B. Nestler, M.D., medical coordinator at Overlook Hospital, Summit, NJ, which has had a medical audit program in effect for years and was one of the testing and demonstration sites used in the development of QAP. According to Dr. Nestler, the medical audit program at Overlook hadn't accomplished much toward changing physician behavior there until the hospital began to establish its own criteria. Then length of stay, preadmission testing, use of blood and medications, and other indexes began to change rapidly for some staff members whose practices were shown to be out of line with Overlook's own norms.[7] A medical consultant explained why: "A physician can always find a reason, at least in his own mind, why his methods and results are at variance with somebody else's norm or a standard established by some far-off authority. But when he's shown to be out of step with his own colleagues, he begins to squirm inside, and things begin to happen." Sometimes it isn't even necessary to call his attention to the variances, the consultant said. "It's better all around if the physician makes his own changes on his own initiative." But it doesn't often happen that way. "This is not an easy business," said Dr. Brown. "If what we're really talking about is changing physicians' behavior, that takes a lot of work."

The reason it isn't easy is that physicians don't like to be told what to do and not do, even by their own colleagues. They like it a lot less when the directives come from physicians at a distance, as in a PSRO, and less still in the form of instructions compiled in an impersonal manual or "medical cookbook." But what they like least of all is any indication that something is wrong and needs to be changed if it comes from a nonmedical source, such as a government bureau, for example, or, less odious but only slightly so, the governing board of a hospital. "Only doctors can judge doctors," was the dictum, and everybody believed it and lived by it. Some still do, or try to, but it's getting harder all the time as the paying agencies impose their controls and as medical information technology makes it possible for some judgments, at least, to be applied by anybody who can read and understand figures. If everybody else on the staff is discharging appendectomy patients on the fifth or sixth day but Dr. X's patients stay nine days, or if everybody but Dr. X is using packed cells and he won't use anything but whole blood, the most uncomprehending layman on the board is going to ask, "Why?"

The reason more boards are asking more questions, and not always accepting the easy answers, is not just that they have more information than they used to have or that the paying agencies are demanding more assurances, but chiefly because the courts increasingly are laying responsibility for what happens to patients on the hospital, not just its attending physicians. Every hospital trustee who takes time to read his mail knows what happened in the *Darling* and *Nork* cases and understands that these and other, similar court decisions of recent years have unalterably and significantly changed the nature of trustee responsibility. Actually, there are varying legal interpretations of precisely how and how much the responsibility has changed. The still prevailing view among hospital lawyers is the more moderate interpretation. *Darling* and *Nork* were extreme cases, in this view: In *Darling*, the hospital personnel, because of the harsh facts, that is, obvious negligence of the attending physician over a period of two weeks, had a duty to intervene; and in *Nork*, where the court noted that the physician admitted performing 36 unnecessary operations over a period of nine years, the governing board had a duty to purge the hospital of what one legal commentator described as "an infamous butcher."

But the broad imposition of hospital liability for all the acts of all the independent physicians practicing within its facilities foreseen by some medicolegal authorities following the *Darling* decision has not occurred. "The few courts which have read *Darling* to impose liability upon the hospital for isolated incidents of malpractice by an independent physician appear to require a kind of gross negligence by the hospital before they will hold the hospital liable," said Joel D. Cunningham, a hospital attorney practicing in the state of Washington.[8] "Nonetheless, the courts have accepted the peripheral holding of *Darling* that there is a hospital duty to investigate and review the general competence of independent physicians. However, the doctrines in the various jurisdictions regarding the hospital-physician relationship are diverse and often completely unrelated. Thus care must be exercised when the results of a court in one jurisdiction are transferred to another jurisdiction, even though the factual setting may be identical."

Most of the commentators who have written and lectured on the subject share the view that *Darling* and *Nork* and a few similar decisions in other jurisdictions constitute a warning to governing boards that gross negligence and rampant incompetence will not be tolerated and that delegation of responsibility to the medical staff is not something that can be declared and thereafter periodically solemnly reaffirmed but not otherwise disinterred. Notable authorities like Don Harper Mills of Los Angeles, a physician-lawyer who lectures at the University of Southern California School of Medicine, and John R. Heher of Trenton, NJ, former chairman of the AHA's Committee on Hospital Governing Boards, emphasize to their clients and audiences that delegation is by no means to be considered a legal act of absolution, handing the total responsibility for patient care on to the medical staff. Far from it, what are handed on to the staff in the process of delegation are the authority to act in matters of medical care and the *primary* responsibility for medical results. But the board retains the ultimate responsibility for patient care, as it does for management, and it also retains a measure of authority, such as authority for approval of appointments and privileges, and for establishing the terms of staff accountability to the board for the proper discharge of *its* responsibility. Thus, in the sensible performance of its retained duties the board is obliged to keep informed of how, and how well, the staff is performing its duties.

Before the problems attendant on keeping informed can be examined, however, it is necessary to consider that there is quite another legal interpretation of the meaning of the *Darling* and *Nork* decisions. This is the belief that in these and other opinions, the courts are articulating a new doctrine of "hospital corporate responsibility" or, as some have chosen to describe it, a new concept of hospital liability for "corporate negligence." Among those who have seen the new doctrine emerging and, in effect, fusing the hospital corporation and its medical staff into a single entity are John F. Horty, Pittsburgh hospital attorney, and David S. Rubsamen of Berkeley, CA, who, like Dr. Mills, is both a physician and a lawyer and is recognized as an authority on professional liability. In Dr. Rubsamen's opinion, the doctrine of corporate responsibility promises far more stringent controls on medical practice than are contemplated in PSRO and utilization review regulations.

Reviewing the recent decisions in an article in the *New England Journal of Medicine*, Dr. Rubsamen quoted the California judge in the *Nork* case as having stated: "The hospital by virtue of its custody of the patient owed him a duty of care; this duty includes the obligation to protect him from acts of malpractice by his independently retained physician who is a member of the hospital staff if the hospital knows, or has reason to know, or should have known, that such acts were likely to occur."[9] It is important to realize that the duty of care owed by the hospital implies a particular standard, Dr. Rubsamen pointed out. "The common-law method for resolving due-care standards, of course, is to submit such questions to a jury," he said. "Only if the facts developed during trial leave no room for reasonable men to differ will the judge decide the issue without permitting it to reach the jury." And a jury might readily see negligence and corporate liability in acts a lot less flagrant than those involved in the *Darling* and *Nork* cases, he suggested. In any jurisdiction where the corporate responsibility rule either exists or seems likely to develop, he recommended that "regarding non-specialist care, except where the physician's competence is at a high level, a system of mandatory consultation for all life-threatening illnesses and for those carrying a risk of serious residual disability should be created."

Dr. Rubsamen noted that recent decisions in Georgia, Nevada, Arizona, Montana, and Missouri have adopted the corporate responsibility concept either in whole or in part. In Nevada, for example, the Supreme Court defined a hospital's responsibility "to create a workable system whereby the medical staff of the hospital continually reviews and evaluates the quality of care being rendered within the institution. The hospital's role is no longer limited to the furnishing of physical facilities and equipment where a physician treats his private patients and practices his profession in his own individualized manner."[10] In Arizona, "The hospital had assumed the duty of supervising the competence of its staff doctors. The department of surgery was acting for and on behalf of the hospital in fulfilling this duty, and if the department was negligent in not taking any action against [the defendant physician] or recommending to the board of trustees that action be taken, then the hospital would also be negligent."[11]

The states that have approved the concept of corporate responsibility are still very much in the minority, Dr. Rubsamen acknowledged. Elsewhere, "traditional law regards the physician as an independent contractor for whom the hospital administration cannot be directly responsible. So the final vote is not in. But one need only recall the Supreme Court's 1972 decision in favor of abortion to recognize how quickly a judicial decision can cut through a social issue and give society a new direction with regard to it. The moment hospital corporate responsibility is established in a jurisdiction all cases that come to trial after that time will be governed by it. It is my guess that most major jurisdictions will adopt the hospital corporate responsibility rule. Therefore, strengthening of hospital peer review and quality control, where necessary, is immediately advisable." In a lecture to a group of hospital executives in California, Dr. Rubsamen offered a last word. "Times are changing," he said. "The burden is now on the hospital to have a system of consultation, peer review and medical care evaluation, and to make the system work."

Actually, the varying interpretations of the *Darling* and *Nork* decisions differ mainly in the legal concepts involved and in their assessments of the degree of negligence that is required to carry liability beyond the independently practicing physician to the hospital corporation, that is, to the administration and the governing board. In any case, the burden is on the administration and governing board to make certain that the medical staff is discharging its delegated responsibilities. This can be done only if the administration and the governing board know what is going on.

In this as in so many other aspects of the management of hospital affairs, the method and content and reliability of the communication system can determine whether the board is really doing its job or simply going through the motions and hoping for the best.

There have always been wild variations in the reporting practices of hospitals. In well-organized teaching institutions, the presence of students and full-time chiefs of the clinical services and the demands of internship and residency approval programs have required detailed reporting of clinical results within the departments and within the medical faculties and staffs. What went along to the administration and governing board was determined for the most part by JCAH requirements, which in the past were more concerned with the existence of records than with their content or detail, and also by local interest and custom. Monthly statistical summaries usually sufficed; few board members gave these more than cursory attention. Problems that couldn't be resolved within the staff, that is, those that threatened either cost or publicity, or both, came to board members via discussions in joint conference or professional relations committee meetings, or, in extremis, due-process sessions of the executive committee. Some administrators who got inquisitive about details of medical affairs got information, and some got the knife, depending on the disposition of the doctors and the diplomatic skills of the administrators involved.

In less well organized hospitals the channels of communication were about the same, but it was thin soup all the way up the line, for the most part, because not so much information was generated within the departments. Administration was required to keep a score of attendance at staff meetings and medical record delinquencies; administrators and super board members always knew about the soft spots, and JCAH requirements were a club that could be counted on to speed up the laggards and weed out the recidivists. The system, such as it was, met the relaxed demands of the time for board attention to credentials, privileges, records, and discipline, and, as new techniques like tissue committees and medical audits were evolved to meet the progressively more exacting requirements coming from within the profession, these could be handled and, if asked for, reported to the board, usually in about as much detail as it was considered appropriate for the board to know.

Now all this has been changed, as we have seen, by the demands of the paying agencies, the consumer representatives in and out of government, the courts, and most of all by the communications technology that makes detailed reporting of medical results as easy as QAP. But minds don't change as fast as technology does, and some boards still have some difficulty in finding out what is going on and is now considered to be their business to know.

The JCAH interpretation of its new standard says that the "general findings of and specific recommendations from" evaluation studies must be reported to the chief executive and the governing body, an artfully unexplicit requirement that inclines with the times toward more detailed communication than has prevailed in the past, but still leaves room for anybody who wants, and some do, to keep the lid on. Thus a lawyer who is a trustee of two hospitals in a Western city and has become thoroughly sensitized to his responsibility for knowing the medical score is provoked because he isn't regularly receiving the professional activity and medical audit (PAS-MAP) reports for his hospitals. "We ought to get that information," he said, "but so far it hasn't come to either board. As far as I'm concerned, I'm going to insist on having it in both cases, because I think this is one of the things we can get into. I've been told that the information can easily be misinterpreted by a layman. Maybe so—I haven't seen it yet, so I don't know. I can understand that the fact that your figures are normal doesn't mean that you're good, or that you are necessarily bad if you happen to fall outside the normal range. I can buy that, but I'd like to know where we stand. Especially, I want to know where we are outside the norms. I'm not looking to find trouble, I just want to know the answer to the questions: 'Could this be a weak spot?' 'How do we find out?' Let's have the answers, the way we get them as directors of corporations when we look at the balance sheets and the income and expense statements. When the signals are there, you'd better take a good look."

The trustee was asked if physicians on the medical staffs had actually opposed having board members see the PAS-MAP reports, and he said he really couldn't answer the question. "The reports are new here," he explained, "I bring it up and they say, 'Well, we're just analyzing the information.' This was six weeks ago, and I still haven't seen anything. Obviously there is some hesitancy about bringing these reports to the board. I'm not going to make a judgment yet whether this is deliberate. I'm willing to wait a bit longer. I'd like to give them every opportunity in the world first to find out exactly where they stand, and give them a chance to get all the answers if anything seems out of line. But the boards are going to have to insist, finally, because I don't know of anything else right now that will give us this information, and of course under present conditions we are responsible, and could be liable. I don't know that it's right for the board to be responsible, but whether it is or it isn't, there it is, and we're going to have to live with it. Again, it's like a corporation board. Sometimes we have to force the management to disgorge the information necessary to reach a conclusion. Otherwise you have people evaluating themselves, and you never get a right answer on that one, because I'm always going to make myself look pretty darn good to myself, and so are you. So is everybody else."*

The existence of pockets of resistance to change such as the medical staffs reported here shouldn't be interpreted to mean that doctors everywhere have drawn their wagons into a circle with their quality evaluations inside and are constantly on guard to repel the encircling barbarians. Inevitably, it is the problem hospitals, like the problem schools and industries and cities, that invite attention and so are the ones that are investigated and reported as a necessary first step toward resolving the problems. Inevitably, too, such reports are seen by some as indications either that conflicts are breaking out all over the place or that "the press never reports all the good things we do," and this is as true of conflicts in hospital-physician relations as it is of vandalism in the schools, mismanagement in industry, and crime in the cities. Thus the episodes reported here and their counterparts elsewhere, taken altogether, constitute the exception, not the rule. There couldn't be a hospital anywhere in which there haven't been disagreements between the board of trustees and the medical staff, or the staff and the administration, or all three. But hospitals, like families, either resolve their disagreements or learn to live with them; if this were not the case, both institutions would long since have vanished.

One method of communication that has been successful not only in solving problems of board-staff jurisdiction but in identifying disagreements as they surface and preventing them from rising to combat level is the practice of having

---

*This trustee also had a word to say about what used to be considered the toughest problem boards ever had to face in the area of medical jurisdiction: the need to cut down privileges or terminate staff appointments. With increasingly better methods of monitoring patient care and requirements for quality assessment, however, he expected that staff awareness of lapses would be improved, offenders would either be turned around or weeded out at an earlier stage, and fewer cases would have to be referred to the board for drastic action. "However, we've had a few," he said. "We had a surgeon doing too many operations that couldn't be justified. It was terrible, and we finally just dropped him. He was entitled to due process, of course, but he knew he was guilty and never requested a hearing. It was a clear-cut case of abuse. We found out later that he'd been dropped from two other staffs, so actually it was a failure of the credentials system, and we learned something from it. In a few other cases the staff has come to us and said, 'You've got to support us,' and we, in turn, have said to them, 'Okay, now we have to depend on you to be willing, if anything happens, to come to court and testify and stay with it. If you believe it and stay with your position, we'll act for you.' And they have, and we have."

physician members of board committees and trustee members of medical staff committees. Like the appointment of physicians to hospital board and executive committee membership, the appointment of medical staff members to such board committees as professional relations, planning, joint conference, and accreditation has become commonplace, and physician members are also being increasingly named on finance, public relations, personnel, and other committees as a seemingly desirable step toward involving physicians in management and making them more aware of the impact their patient care decisions have on every phase of hospital operations. "Committees serve as an excellent vehicle to educate the members of the committee about the interaction and interdependence of trustees, medical staff members, and members of the administrative staff," said Madison B. Brown, M.D., AHA senior vice-president, in a memorandum to the AHA's Committee on Physicians.[12]

Up to now, however, the reciprocating appointment of trustees to medical staff committees hasn't kept pace, though some hospitals have initiated the practice, apparently with satisfactory results. But as Dr. Brown said, "Medical staffs have long looked upon their committees as being peer committees composed exclusively of members of the medical staff. Sometimes this has meant that the chief executive officer was not a member or a member ex officio of the executive committee of the medical staff." In this as in other traditional hospital practices, the external pressures are having an effect, and, according to Dr. Brown, "A new appraisal of the membership of some of the committees of the medical staff seems justified. If one accepts the premise that governance, management, and decision making in the health care institution involves, depending on the problem, at times members of one peer group and at other times the combination of trustees, administrative staff, and medical staff, then we can look more objectively at trustee representation on appropriate medical staff committees."

In fact, Dr. Brown pointed out, a number of the medical staff executive committee functions as these are commonly described in staff bylaws* might readily be expedited by trustee representation on the committee. "As the committee evaluates the issues and formulates its responses and recommendations, wouldn't it be valuable to have a knowledgeable trustee or trustees participate in these deliberations?" he asked. "The trustees would then be better informed and become more sensitive to medical staff policy and philosophy," he suggested. Moreover, such participation shouldn't be looked on as lay domination or inter-

---

*Dr. Brown mentioned specifically recommendations to the board on staff appointments and privileges, accreditation, planning, medical administration, and matters concerned with the overall quality and efficiency of medical care.

ference, since the committee membership would always remain predominantly physicians, and nonphysician members, like administrator members, would not vote on any matters involving medical judgments. For much the same reasons, trustee members of staff committees having to do with quality assurance, accreditation, utilization review, and medical audit, all now involving trustee responsibility, would afford further opportunities for improved effectiveness, and, in fact, the AHA's QAP manual recommends that the staff's quality assurance program committee should be multidisciplinary in its representation, including trustee members.

Finally, Dr. Brown argued, trustee representation on the staff credentials committee would appear to make functional as well as educational sense. "Recommendations for the privileges to be granted members of the medical staff and changes in privileges are delicate and sensitive responsibilities of this committee," he acknowledged in his memorandum. "Too often, the medical staff looks upon the function of this committee as involving only medical peer judgment. However, there are other concerns in which the counsel of a trustee could be most helpful, as, for example, the physician's reputation in the community outside the medical community and the opinion of other trustees in hospitals where the physician has staff privileges." In summary, Dr. Brown concluded, "Any approach to the involvement of trustees on committees of the medical staff will come as a new venture to most hospitals. Recognition of the fact that several committees of the medical staff do require other than physician representatives, and particularly the chief executive officer or his representative, provides the opportunity also to include trustee representatives."

Thus we come to the key consideration in board-staff communications and, in fact, everything else having to do with the board-staff relationship: the position and function of the administrator, president, or, in the newly popular terminology, chief executive officer—by any title obviously the pivotal person in the whole complex. Again, in order to understand how he got into the quicksand, it is necessary to consider where he came from. In the distant past, which is to say up until the complexities introduced by specialization, technology, and prepayment began to emerge in the years preceding World War II, there were in the main just two types of hospital administrator.

The director or general superintendent of the major teaching or charity hospital was almost invariably a physician, often one who still practiced medicine part of the time, and the unquestioned commander-in-chief of the entire institution and everything and everybody in it, including the physicians. He met with the board of trustees as an equal and did most of the talking at board meetings, excepting only when the subject of the discussion was finance, which he was glad to leave largely if not wholly in the hands of the trustees.

The other type of administrator was just as plainly not a leader but a follower, if not a servant, of the board and staff. Sometimes this was a nurse who ascended to her position through the nursing hierarchy but remained for all her eminence and responsibility in her traditional role as the doctors' handmaiden. In church-affiliated hospitals, the administrator was often a member of the religious order or a retired clergyman, hard-working and dedicated to patient care, but again trained to regard the doctor's wish as a command and the trustee's beneficence and knowledge of money matters as less than divine, but just barely. A few administrators, including some of the best, had worked their way up from the cashier's window and the business office; some were retired businessmen or physicians, and a few were businessmen or physicians who had not so much retired as failed at their initial endeavors, and whose appointment provided a clue to the regard for the position that prevailed generally among the hospital trustees and practicing physicians of their time.

That time is long gone. The first of the graduate university programs in hospital administration was established in the mid-1930s; as the complexities of the management assignment became more and more evident during the war and postwar years, demand created supply and the programs multiplied. Study commissions on education for hospital administration in 1948 and 1954 contributed to the refinement of the educational process, and for the past 20 years, at least, the hospital administrator who has not been trained for his responsibilities in one of the univeristy programs or by related and equivalent professional or business training and experience has been a rarity and doomed to early extinction, like the blue whale. And yet, just as the hospital itself still bears vestiges of its early function as charitable and religious asylum for the infirm poor, traces of the years of servitude of his professional antecedents may remain and get in the way of an effective peer relationship between the administrator and the medical staff. The delicacy of the position is implicit in hospital organization charts, which nearly always show the link between the administrator and the staff as a dotted line, and a dotted line on an organization chart can mean only one thing: "Don't ask!"

While the modern hospital administrator is as different from the handmaiden as the computer is from the abacus, the change has been accomplished within the span of a single generation; when the senior members of today's medical staffs were in their internships, the administrator was somebody who was told what to do by the chief of service. Thus it isn't surprising that those who think it should be the other way around today are having a hard time making the idea stick. Foremost among those who are trying is the American College of Hospital Administrators, whose board of governors recommended, in response to an invitation from the commission to comment, that the JCAH standards should be revised to make the chief executive officer accountable to the governing authority for all functions of the hospital, including medical, nursing, technical, and general services. "The function of governance is judgmental and deliberative," said the ACHA publication, commenting on the recommendation. [13] "Therefore, the governing authority appoints a chief executive responsible for the performance of all functions of the institution and accountable to the governing authority. The chief executive, as the operating head of the organization, is responsible for all functions, including a medical staff, nursing division, technical division, and general services division, which will be necessary to assure the quality of patient care." In the ACHA construct, the governing authority in consultation with the chief executive and a committee of the medical staff selects a physician for appointment as chief of staff, "whose function is to assure the governing authority and its chief executive that the expected quality of medical care is achieved." In the ACHA organization chart, the chief executive sits in the same box with the governing authority, and the lines connecting them with the chief of staff, medical executive committee, chiefs of service, and staff are not dotted.

Another outspoken advocate of administrative authority is the Catholic Hospital Association. In a 1974 publication entitled *Guidelines on the Roles and Relationships of Board, Chief Executive Officer, and Medical Staff of Catholic Hospital and Long-Term Care Facilities*, the CHA specified that it should be the function of the chief executive officer, among other things, "to establish mechanisms for exacting accountability from the medical staff organization and to act as the official channel of contact between the board and the medical staff organization." [14] Then, in an introductory paragraph preceding the medical staff guidelines, the publication stated: "It is essential for physicians to understand the over-all process of management and to participate in this process. Through this understanding the physicians will recognize that through the chief executive officer, they are accountable to the ultimate authority of the board of trustees for the practice of medicine in the institution. The board must rely on accepted management principles for holding the medical staff accountable and must make sure that the chief executive officer applies these principles in his dealings with the medical staff in the same way he does when dealing with every other component of the organization."

In an exegesis of the Catholic Hospital Association position at a conference of hospital trustees, administrators, and physicians, Paul Donnelly, Ph.D., CHA vice-president, said that "continuing confusion in the relationships between physicians, administrators, and boards makes hospitals sitting ducks to any outside marksman who wants to take potshots that result in even greater external regulation. Hospitals and physicians are without a united front, and even the fundamental understanding of where responsibility lies and who has a legitimate right to exercise authority. We cannot hope to address these complexities with outdated structures which don't stand the test of solid management principles."[15]

The boards, with few exceptions, are made up of people with full-time commitments in other walks of life, Dr. Donnelly said, and "because of this attribute of our voluntary boards of trustees, it is essential that there be someone to act for the board in a full-time capacity, as its agent. It is also essential that this person be vested with the responsibility for the total operation of the hospital and be accountable to the board for the utilization of its resources. If the chief executive officer does not have the medical resources included among the things for which he is responsible, he has one hand tied behind his back, the same as if he had no authority in the financial area or no authority for personnel. The physician component of the hospital is the most essential, and the chief executive officer must have authority to deal in this area if he is going to be effective in carrying out his responsibility. Also, being part-time, the board is ill equipped to have more than one person responsible to it."

But the board doesn't delegate all its authority to the executive, Dr. Donnelly was careful to point out. Necessarily it retains a "package of reserved powers" for staff appointments, and to make certain, for example, that the executive has developed satisfactory systems for involving physicians in decision making, just as it sets limits on the executive's authority to make major expenditures. Like all the rest of us, he suggested, physicians would be happiest if they could do just what they wanted to do, and "what we need to develop are systems which approach that as nearly as possible, yet which recognize the constraints an organization sets on the practice of medicine in the hospital, which is in fact different from the practice of medicine in the physician's own office. We need to provide a formal structure within the total institutional organization whereby physicians can participate in the policy-making and planning process in an organized fashion. As the physician sees and accepts his role in this process, it should overcome a great many of the fears physicians have that 'we are going to be run by a dictator who is going to shove decisions down our throats.' I think we can overcome a great amount of that kind of fear and still maintain the authority delegation patterns that I have described. Without full appreciation of these dimensions, we'll have to settle for less than the excellence that is possible and that is being demanded by society, and we'll have to be content to deal with the same problems that were bugging us 20 and 30 years ago. Public confidence in our private health system is at stake."

While it is likely that many if not most hospital trustees and administrators, not to mention physicians, would throw their hats in the air and cheer unrestrainedly if they had to deal only with the same problems that were bugging them 20 or 30 years ago, not many outside the Catholic Hospital Association, and not by any means all of them inside CHA, would agree that the only route to improved public confidence in the health system is through the precedence of administrative over medical staff authority. In fact, given the sensitivity of most physicians today about encroachments on their independence by laws, regulations, court decisions, and consumer organizations of all kinds, attempts to introduce changes in the hospital authority structure, except as they arise inevitably as required quality assurance measures are initiated and as both physicians and administrators are advanced to membership on hospital boards, could be expected in many cases to result in disputes that might readily be destructive of public confidence.

The JCAH standard on quality of professional services and an AHA policy statement on governance of health care institutions approved by the Association's House of Delegates in 1974 are no less insistent than ACHA and CHA that the board of trustees is ultimately responsible for professional service, as for everything else, but the standard requires only that the staff shall report to the governing board *and*, not *through*, the chief executive officer, and the AHA guidelines statement defines the acts of management of the governing board as "delegation of authority and the sharing of responsibility and accountability with the chief executive officer and the medical staff for delivery of high-quality health care services; effective, efficient, and economical utilization of the institution's resources and services; and full execution of operating policy. Delegation of authority for the operation of the institution to the chief executive officer is essential to achievement of effective management. . . . His effectiveness requires that the governing board carefully delineate his authority, responsibility, and accountability and recognize that he is the person ultimately responsible to the board for the total operation of the hospital."[16]

Thus the policies of ACHA, CHA, and AHA are congruent, if not identical, but the AHA guidelines, unlike the others, comprehend the dotted lines, which is how the real world works. John Alexander McMahon, AHA president, explained why. "Now more than ever, the hospital has need for a chief executive officer who can coordinate the efforts and skills of *all* the different groups in the hospital and who can see that board policy is carried out," he said in the AHA's magazine *Trustee* early in 1975.[17]

"However, no matter how many organization policies, rules, and regulations are established, the question of human relations remains. In decision making, the physician may find this the most difficult area in which to proceed. For the most part, the physician is used to one-to-one relationships in which he is the authority. He is not used to the dynamics of an organized social setting in which a variety of persons have their own views. As the physician's role in institutional decision making is broadened, it must always be kept in mind that from his point of view the central issues are those directly involving a patient. Everything else may at times seem secondary or trivial.

"The hospital needs a chief executive officer whose primary concern is improvement of the process whereby health care services are delivered to the public. As he works to create a healthy working environment between the governing board, the medical staff, and the other hospital departments, he will have to call upon his skills as a manager, a teacher, an interpreter, and a diplomat.

"I believe that increased involvement by the government, by the courts, and by the consumer will be more than enough impetus for us to sit down at our individual hospitals to reassess, to analyze, and to plan for the future. At no time in history have all sectors of the hospital team been more willing and more ready to thrust aside their adversary roles and join forces in a collective effort. We must seize this moment and build upon it. I am confident we shall."

Much as they might like to see clear lines of authority established throughout the hospital, in accordance with accepted principles of management, trustees increasingly understand that the position of the physician in private practice sets conditions for executive and governing authority that do not exist in the management of other enterprises. They decide to wait a bit longer before insisting on having the information, and they back off, instead of blowing the lid off, when they encounter delays in implementing decisions. They have the unquestioned authority to insist and to act if they wish, and in most cases much the same authority is delegated to the administrator by policy and bylaw provisions, but except in cases of clear dereliction they keep the club in the closet and let the medical staff machinery work, even when it grinds slowly. They may do a little Indian wrestling from time to time, but, like the smart administrator, they know how to treat molehills as molehills.

7. YOU CAN'T DO ANYTHING WITHOUT MONEY

"I hate to hear it called a not-for-profit business," said John Sturgis, the banker turned hospital executive, "because you know it gives the man in the street the idea that we aren't supposed to make money in the hospital business. So you do make a profit, and of course there's only one place it goes, and that is right back into services in one form or another. The list of things we need and want every year far exceeds our profit. Unfortunately, in the accounting system we aren't allowed to show unmet needs. We can only footnote them, and we're going to have to do a better job of showing the public that we're always working against a list of millions of dollars of needed equipment and facilities. You can't do anything without money. Sometimes I get in trouble with some of the older directors here who really in some funny ways were more comfortable with a deficit, from a philosophical point of view."

It is doubtful that there can be many hospital trustees today, whatever their seniority, who are getting very much philosophical comfort from their hospitals' deficits. Uniquely among large city teaching institutions, Sturgis's Northwestern Memorial is located in a comfortable urban residential area and so is relatively free of the demands that create deficits for these hospitals elsewhere as urban populations swarm in their outpatient and emergency departments, requiring services nobody is going to pay for.

For years, hospitals met these deficits the only way they could: by charging paying patients more to cover the cost of those who paid less. But the paying agencies have been relentlessly squeezing out consideration of any costs not related to services for their own beneficiaries. Rate setting, or, in the more polite terminology, rate reviewing, commissions have been established in a dozen or more jurisdictions and are obviously coming in others. It is still possible to get philanthropic and community support for facility expansion and improvement, but it is harder all the time to get operating deficits paid this way as the impression grows that Medicare, Medicaid, and local health and welfare agencies pay for everybody who can't pay for himself. This comes close to being true, in a way, but it leaves completely out of consideration the critical fact that none of the agencies pays the whole cost, and some of them, especially in the case of outpatient services, pay as little as half the cost.

Thus in New York City, which in 1975 appeared to lead the nation in every kind of financial trouble known to man, the United Hospital Fund reported that its 55 voluntary hospital members had lost $85 million in the last year, an estimated $50 million of it on ambulatory services. The fund's annual report said that two hospitals had closed, two others were in receivership, and 14 more were "technically insolvent," receiving some form of fiscal artificial respiration.[1] As these conditions became known, some relief was forthcoming from some of the paying agencies, but a few hospitals had already started to curtail services. In New York and other cities, obviously, only major changes in reimbursement policies, particularly for ambulatory care, would provide a real solution.

Financial pressures came from all over. As unemployment mounted, some workers and their families lost their hospitalization insurance and postponed care, depressing hospital occupancies; others couldn't pay for care that couldn't be delayed, depressing hospital cash registers. Insurance companies and prepayment plans tightened their claims policies and took longer to pay. The malpractice squeeze and resultant "doctors' strikes" caused further losses. Employers contributing to their employees' health insurance became increasingly critical about services and costs. In Phoenix, Motorola, Inc., publicly castigated hospital management for alleged extravagant practices. The points at issue were resolved, finally, but the dispute did not improve public confidence in hospital financial management. Other nationwide employers started making comparisons of their employees' health care costs in various parts of the country, a seemingly prudent measure that nevertheless added to the confusion when, inevitably, Washington's apples were compared to Florida's oranges. The National Commission on Productivity and Work Quality labored and came up with a laundry list of recommendations for hospitals that touched all the familiar bases, from management engineering to shared service, raising once again the question of whether the usefulness of such commissions in calling public attention to ways existing practices can be improved isn't cancelled out by the erroneous impression they leave that the obvious things are newly discovered and not already being done. What with one thing and another, the inescapable obligation of the trustee to ensure the survival of the enterprise wasn't getting any easier.

Why not? As in so many elements of hospital practice that confound observers by seeming to fall outside the boundaries of acceptable business thought, the reason is more historical than logical. In a wryly humorous paper presented at a state hospital association meeting in 1974 and winningly entitled "Financing toward Bankruptcy," Harold Hinderer, financial adviser to the hospitals operated by the Daughters of Charity and a respected authority on hospital financial management, traced a large measure of the chronic underfunding that is responsible for so many hospital problems today back to a policy established by agreement between hospitals and Blue Cross in 1953, when the accounting concepts and practices of hospitals were still emerging from the penumbra of their charitable antecedents.[2] A principle of payment for hospital care included in the agreement stipulated at that time that bad debts, courtesy allowances, and the unpaid costs of care of the indigent were to be regarded as deductions from earned income and not included as reimbursable cost. In order to understand how such a policy, long since discarded and plainly seen as crippling, if not suicidal, could ever have been solemnly considered and approved by thoughtful hospital leaders, it is necessary to remember that Blue Cross at that time was still closely identified with hospitals; bad debts, courtesy discounts, and free care to the needy were regarded as sacred obligations of local community charities and philanthropies, among which both hospitals and Blue Cross Plans were proud to be counted; half or more of all hospital patients paid their own bills at the hospitals' published rates; it was accepted practice, understood by patients as well as hospitals, for such rates to include an allocation to free care; capital funding was seeded by public Hill-Burton grants but provided for the most part still by philanthropic, public, and corporate beneficence; and anybody who had predicted that within 25 years 90 percent of all hospital revenues would be coming from contracting agencies via reimbursable cost formulations, and most of the capital funds from the money market at the going rate, would have been considered a dangerous maniac. Depreciation was considered by all but the most advanced thinkers as a way to safeguard the charitable image; as one hospital board president used to say every year in his annual report, which always showed a small operating surplus and a deficit after depreciation, "We are wearing out our buildings in service to the community." Everybody was doing it.

By the time Medicare came along in 1966 the thinking about (a) depreciation and (b) working capital, which had been (a) slighted and (b) ignored in the earlier principles, had changed, but government negotiators were not impressed. As Mr. Hinderer noted in his review, their attitude was, "You don't change the rules just because a new team comes into the league." In the Medicare reimbursement formula that emerged, however, the Social Security Administration agreed to an accelerated depreciation option, and a 2 percent "plus factor" (frequently referred to by the delighted but redundant hospital negotiators as an "added plus") was seen as recognition by government that hospitals, like housewives, can't do anything without money.

If it was, it didn't last. In 1969, with Medicare costs exceeding what Social Security Administration actuaries and the Congress had anticipated, the government suddenly and unilaterally eliminated the plus factor and the accelerated depreciation option, and when the federal administration initiated its Economic Stabilization Program in 1971, the health industry, and especially hospitals, were confronted with more rigid controls than were imposed on all but one or two other industries. Explaining the reasons this happened to a group of hospital trustees after all controls had been removed in 1974, Stuart H. Altman, Ph.D., HEW deputy assistant secretary, said it arose from "a sense of an industry out of control," with costs that had been rising at a steeper rate than they had in the rest of the economy. The controls were considered to be temporary measures, he insisted, and there had been no intention to rule out orderly capital accumulation.[3] But Dr. Altman and other government officials had been deaf to AHA arguments that hospital cost rises had been caused for the most part by catch-up wage increases following loss of hospital exemption from the minimum wage provisions of the National Labor Relations Act, and the increases were already leveling off at the time controls were established. The attitude of some government officials, at least, was on display when a representative of the federal Cost of Living Council answered a question at a hospital conference during the ESP years. The administrator of a small institution in the rural South whose request for approval of an increase had been denied asked what kind of hardship would have justified approval of the increase. "Bankruptcy," said the COLC agent. "Well, that's a hardship," the administrator acknowledged.[4]

Obviously, the answer to the question was not intended to be taken literally but only to emphasize that government policy as applied to the financial management of hospitals would be hard line, with minimum tolerance for deviations. It's still that way. At another point in Dr. Altman's 1974 meeting with the hospital trustees, he said, "We have to change the incentive system in hospital care. There is general agreement that the retroactive reimbursement system tends to lead to excesses over time, bringing pressure for regulatory controls. Ultimately the responsiblity for controls has to be yours, but without a blank check. We have to keep regulation at a minimum and change incentives by means of prospective reimbursement."

Under this method, the rate of payment is agreed on in periodic advance negotiations between the institution and the paying agency, and thereafter the institution is penalized for cost overruns but retains an agreed share of any savings that may be realized; this presumably provides a financial incentive for efficiency. One trustee objected that the method would, in fact, reward the hospital that had been inefficient in the past, since the initial rate would have to be related to historical cost, and the hospital that had been efficiently operated would have a harder time earning the incentive margins. "We have to start where we are," Dr. Altman said. "We can't start from scratch. The need is to minimize inequality and not hurt those we want to help. Efficient managers will find a way to live with the system, whatever it is, and inefficient managers will still be inefficient. It isn't ever going to be possible to design a payment system that doesn't have some inequalities."

The American Hospital Association has seen prospective reimbursement as offering a promising opportunity to meet hospital financial requirements and urged its member institutions to aid in the development of demonstration projects. "Payments based on prospectively determined rates have very real opportunities for improvement in meeting the objectives of public accountability, predictability, and preservation of institutional autonomy," said a statement approved by the Association's House of Delegates in 1970. The statement included detailed guidelines for determining rates based on hospital size, scope of services, utilization, location, and other considerations, and for designing a prospective payment system that would provide for emergency adjustments, periodic review, and appeal procedures. In addition to the AHA, several state and regional hospital organizations have been working with the Social Security Administration, Blue Cross, and other payers in prospective payment demonstrations aimed at developing a payment system that will provide appropriate incentives and at the same time protect the interests of both the paying agencies and the institutions providing the services. Medicaid and Blue Cross payments are already established on a prospective basis in a number of states.

The guidelines for prospective payment systems were approved by the AHA as part of a plan for implementing its *Statement on the Financial Requirements of Health*

Care Institutions and Services, which had been adopted in 1969. The statement was developed over a four-year period of study and discussion that was initiated during the Medicare rate negotiations, when it became apparent that the 1953 principles and a succession of later revisions and modifications of the Association's policies on payment and reimbursement had not adequately identified all the financial requirements of hospitals and other health care institutions. "The passage of Public Law 89-97 [Medicare and Medicaid] underscored the fundamental weaknesses in health care financing," said the introduction to the statement. "This governmental program assumed the burden for the payment of health care bills of a large segment of the population but explicitly renounced any obligation to share in the meeting of the total needs of our health care system, except as that system met the needs of the program beneficiaries."

It is the basic assumption of the AHA statement and the policy that it articulates that all contracting agencies must recognize the total community services obligations of the providers of service. "This statement sets forth a set of guidelines for a program to overcome the financial shortcomings that have plagued health care institutions for a long time," said an introductory paragraph. "It states that all purchasers of care must share in the financial requirements of institutions providing that care. Financial requirements, differentiated from costs, are described as those resources necessary not only to meet current operating needs, but sufficient to permit replacement of physical plant, expansion of services, education, research, and a myriad of other obligations heretofore only sporadically recognized and supported by purchasers of care.

"It is recognized that the traditional methods of retrospectively sharing in the cost of capital programs do not adequately finance replacement or new programs and facilities. In the past, this difference was given token recognition, through many mechanisms, such as the addition of an all-inclusive 'plus factor' to cost reimbursement formulas. Many vitally needed health care institutions have never quite been able to meet the community need because of the inherent unpredictability and inequities of this financing system."

In return for the obligation incurred by purchasers to ensure that all the financial needs of the institution are comprehended in the payment formula, the statement continued, the institutions must accept a corollary obligation: "that of assuring the community that the institution's definition of its role is consonant with community need. The planning mechanism must look at the community as a whole and the interrelationships among health care institutions serving that community. The individual institution must have the responsibility and capability to fulfill its community role."

The statement then went on to examine the elements of institutional financial requirements. Current operating needs related to patient care were analyzed as including financial resources for salaries, wages, fringe benefits, services, supplies, maintenance, minor building modification, and applicable taxes; interest on borrowed funds; education and research programs having the appropriate approval; credit losses; and "needs arising from the care of patients who, because of inability to pay, are relieved wholly or in part of financial responsibility for services rendered." Capital needs were defined as including plant capital for the preservation, replacement, and improvement of plant and equipment; expansion needs resulting from population growth, discontinuance of other existing services, and changes in the public concept of health care delivery; and amortization of indebtedness. The need for adequate cash reserves and, in the case of investor-owned hospitals, return on investment were also included among the listed capital needs. The statement also included guidelines for determining and measuring all the listed needs, and then for apportioning the total of institutional requirements appropriately among the beneficiaries of contracting agencies and self-pay patients by accepted cost finding and rate setting methods.

"A complication arises in the apportioning of financial requirements between the two categories: self-pay patients and beneficiaries of contracting agencies," the statement warned. "Both categories share the responsibility for meeting the health care institution's total financial requirements. However, the mechanics of payment may result in the application of different methods of payment. That is, the assessment of the self-pay patient's share is made at the time the service is performed, but the contracting agency's obligation may not be assessed until a later point in time if the method of payment employed has a provision for retroactive adjustment." The statement then outlined the various methods by which equitable apportionments can be determined.

A concluding section examined the reciprocal obligations and responsibilities of health care institutions, contracting agencies, and areawide health planning agencies. "In essence," this said, "the statement declares that the community must provide for proper planning of its health care system and that the health care system must accept, on its part, the community's right to insist on proper planning within that system."

By the time the statement was approved, it was already established that the largest of the contracting agencies, the Social Security Administration, was going to continue to play by the old rules and to change the rules from time to time, usually on the side of further constraints on allowable cost, but not always, as when the initiation of "periodic interim payments" recognized the hospitals' needs for operating cash. As the negotiations have continued on a "win some, lose some" basis, as negotiations always do, unquestionably the hospital position has been strengthened by the statement, which has also aided negotiations with other payers. Especially, the principles and methods set forth in the statement have helped bring about a more orderly and realistic approach to rate setting by hospitals themselves. Contracting agencies and self-supporting and insured patients paying hospital charges are the means by which hospitals must necessarily recover the portion of total financial requirements not provided by cost payers.

At the time the statement was being examined and discussed among AHA's committees and councils prior to its approval by the Association's Board of Trustees and House of Delegates, some hospital trustees had objected that a concept of financial requirements comprehending the interrelationships of institutions and total community needs as seen by planning agencies would intrude on the individual institution's right to determine its own course of action. "If we want to use the money we can raise ourselves to build the facilities and provide the services we think the community should have," the argument ran, "why should we let somebody else decide what we can and can't do?" It was a time when the planning agencies for the most part were at some stage of transition from wholly voluntary groups that were knowledgeable but frequently ineffective to consumer-oriented boards that had government sponsorship and some authority but often no expertise, and so the argument opposing any surrender of hospital autonomy to such groups had a lot of appeal. But the view that prevailed was that areawide planning for health services was not going to disappear; in time it would acquire needed expertise and authority, and hospitals would gain, not lose, by recognizing the legitimacy and necessity of its goals and aiding its development. As we shall see in chapter 8, this is exactly what has been happening in the years since the statement was under consideration.

Meanwhile, also, another development foreseen in the statement has been emerging to highlight the importance of intelligent rate determination as an essential element of hospital financial management. This is the establishment of rate review commissions in the states.

While it is clear that state agencies ultimately will have full authority to require disclosure of hospital financial and operating data, approve budgets and rates, and determine allowable changes in facilities and services, the commissions that had already been established in mid-1975 had a variety of powers. In Massachusetts, the Rate Setting Commission was responsible for establishing prospective rates for state assistance programs and Workmen's Compensation and for approving Blue Cross contracts based on retrospective cost audit. The California Hospital Commission was initiating a statewide system of uniform accounting, reporting, and auditing for public disclosure and would require prospective rates for all classes of purchasers, based on the AHA statement. New Jersey's commissioner of health and commissioner of insurance shared authority for approving Blue Cross and Medicaid rates. The Connecticut Commission on Hospitals and Health Care would have the authority to approve hospital budgets for expense, revenue, and capital funding. The Maryland Health Services Cost Review Commission had instituted a uniform accounting and reporting system, but the Maryland Hospital Association went to court to challenge the commission's interpretation of the law regarding its rate setting authority, and the issue was still in litigation in mid-1975. In an interim decision enjoining the commission from enforcing its assumed authority, the court described a set of guidelines the commission had issued to hospitals as "gobbledygook." Ironically, the Maryland Hospital Association had endorsed the law creating the commission, and the commissioner who sought to freeze hospital rates pending settlement of the dispute was a former hospital administrator.

The American Hospital Association in 1972 had anticipated the trend to state rate regulatory commissions and formulated its own guidelines aimed at making certain as far as possible that the commissions would observe the principles laid down in the *Statement on Financial Requirements of Health Care Institutions and Services*. Assuming that rates would be established prospectively to apportion financial requirements without discrimination among all purchasers of care, the guidelines then considered standards for defining the authority and responsibility of a state commission, its relationship to planning, and the rate review process, including the evaluation of reasonableness, indications for change, the reporting procedure, time considerations, provisions for emergency situations, and the appeal mechanism. Recognizing, as Stuart Altman said, that "we have to start where we are," the AHA proposed that "At the time of the establishment of the commission and the promulgation of its administrative regulations, the rates of all health care institutions then currently offered should be deemed reasonable, adequate, and proper, in the absence of evidence to the contrary; they would thus be constructively approved by the commission. Once approved, rates could be continued in effect unless changes are otherwise ordered or permitted by the commission. Consideration of changes in rates could be initiated either by the institution or by the commission, either by its own initiative or by a valid request on the part of the consuming public."[5]

Some states have chosen to begin the implementation of rate review in a trial or pilot group of institutions prior to taking on full responsibility; others have started with uniform accounting and reporting requirements, with their laws specifying that rate review will be phased in at a later time. "Regardless of the approach used," the AHA said, "full implementation of the rate review and approval process should be approached with due consideration of the importance of developing a sound process as well as meeting the urgency of the timing."

That it isn't going to happen exactly that way is already apparent from the experience in Maryland and, for example, Massachusetts, where the commissions appeared to have reversed the recommended approach, beginning with the assumption of full authority and working backward to figure out the processes and standards. These methods, which are not unknown in other fields regulated by state authority, have caused some hospital trustees to oppose the formation of state commissions and consider that hospital associations invite disaster by lending their support to the movement toward public utility-type regulation by the states. At the other extreme, some health economists, union officials, and other consumer representatives oppose state authority because state commissions tend to become captives of the industries they are supposed to regulate and are thus ineffective as representatives of the public interest.

It seems likely, however, that most trustees, like most hospital administrators and association executives, consider that given the existing degree of public funding, controls are inevitable, and that state authority will probably prove more manageable, and more desirable, than federal authority would be, and the extremes of arbitrary dictatorship by the states, on the one hand, and ineffectual submissiveness, on the other, can probably be avoided.

This was the view expressed in an interview with Henry Gardner, vice-chairman of the board of directors of Northwestern Memorial Hospital in Chicago. As president of a Chicago bank, Mr. Gardner is not unaccustomed to dealing with state and federal authority. "We have many regulations to comply with," he said, "and we have to report to and deal with many different agencies of the government, but we don't have to spend any concentrated amounts of time with it except when they are in here making an examination. The rest of the time we comply with the rules. Sure, there's a cost to us — a fairly high cost, simply keeping up with what comes out of Washington and Springfield — but I don't think it's as concentrated as it is in the hospital field, because it isn't changing so quickly. In the hospital field, there's something new every day. I look at this with mixed feelings, because quite honestly I believe the industry as a whole needs a certain amount of discipline, and philosophically I agree with rate mechanisms and screening of facilities and equipment. Somebody has to do it. I'm still a private enterprise type and mistrust the bureaucratic mechanism to do it right. But to the extent that the industry can't do it, I presume some mechanism has to be brought into being."

Actually, the argument about the desirability of state hospital authority became largely academic anyway at the end of 1974 with passage of the National Health Planning and Resources Development Act, calling for the establishment of state health planning and development agencies. The law (see chapter 8) provides for grants to the states "for the purpose of demonstrating the effectiveness of state agencies regulating rates," and another provision calls for the Secretary of HEW to "establish a uniform system of accounting and statistical reporting for institutional providers of health care, including a uniform system for calculating rates to be charged to health insurers and other payors." It may be several years before the system is in effect in all the jurisdictions, and it may not work very well when it is, and hospital associations and medical societies will continue to seek amendments to some of the provisions that are seen as threatening. But it seems settled that there will be state hospital authorities, and it is likely that states like California, where an experienced hospital administrator is a member of the commission and most of its programs have been worked out with the cooperation of the state hospital association, will be better off in the long run than the states whose hospitals have chosen instead to hide in the bushes and growl.

Whether the ultimate control of rates goes to the state or remains with the individual institution, or whether it is partly one and partly the other, however, the basic instrument of financial management, and hence the exercise of control by the board of trustees, is the budget — a delegated responsibility of administration whose seminal importance requires that the board, or some of its members, had better be involved in, or informed of, budget planning and reporting. "The time has arrived for medical staffs and trustees to realistically come to grips with basic questions of financial planning, financial control, financial reporting, and financial education as these relate to their own hospital operations," said Raymond E. Scroggins, a trustee and member of the executive committee of the board of Deaconess Hospital, Milwaukee. In an article in *Trustee* magazine, Mr. Scroggins suggested that the budget is the obvious and effective means by which the interested groups can get a firm handhold.[6]

The processes of budgeting and using the budget for purposes of control are the same in hospitals as they are in most other businesses, but some differences in the planning and use of budgets are immediately evident. The first of these is a matter of mission. There may be good reasons for the hospital to establish a service that is needed by the community, for example, when prudent budgeting for income and expense would declare the project insane on the face of it, and there are always occasions when service demands or circumstances argue for departures from budgets that have been established and approved on the basis of sound and careful planning. These things can happen in business, of course, but in the hospital the occasions are likely to be more frequent and the reasons for departures more compelling.

Another important difference is that budgeting for revenue is chancier in the hospital than it is in many businesses. In the first place, nobody knows for sure who is going to get sick or hurt and require what services, in what volume, and then there is no sales manager who can be exhorted to beat the bushes for orders if revenues fall below expectations, and fired if he doesn't produce. There are no advertising programs that can be stepped up to bring customers out from behind the trees when sales lag. This is not to say that the process is entirely random. The closest thing the hospital has to a sales force is the medical staff. Careful budgeting comprehends continuing analysis of the age and composition of the staff, the patterns of medical practice, the composition and movement of the population, economic circumstances of the community, and the availability of services in other institutions. When all these factors are carefully considered and appropriate weight given to historical experience, it is possible to estimate hospital revenues with about the same tolerances that can be expected in business. A factor that favors hospitals is the fact that the incidence of disease and injury in large population groups over time can be predicted a lot more precisely than anybody can foretell how the public may respond to a new brand of deodorant or sugar-coated whatsies. Marketing is not an exact science, to begin with, and most businesses are susceptible to some circumstance that may make a mockery of the budget, the way a scientific breakthrough or an epidemic may affect the hospital.

As in any established business, budgeting for expense leans heavily on the historical record, with adjustments for known and anticipated changes. The methods for identifying cost centers and handling undistributed expenses, for involving department managers in expense budgeting and making them accountable for performance, and for handling exceptions are not substantially different in the hospital. More often than not, when differences do arise they are attributable to the unique position of physicians in the determination of how personnel and material resources are used. The only possible way the effects of this circumstance can be foreseen and modified is either by getting physicians involved in budget planning or systematically keeping them informed as budgets are developed and experience unfolds during the budget period. This won't solve all the problems, but most hospitals have found that it cuts down the incidence of surprises and collisions.

The introduction of computers has made the reporting process faster and easier. As Mr. Scroggins described it, "Accounting and computer techniques can provide good information. However, as the material is made available for study by the administration, the board, and the medical staff, some questions must be asked: Is the hospital making the best use of all space and equipment? Is the hospital taking advantage of the best purchasing opportunities? Is the hospital utilizing employees to maximum advantage? The routine questions are similar to those every manager must face. Additionally, however, the hospital's administration and board are confronted with problems they cannot control without the cooperation of the medical staff."

At a recent conference of corporate directors, Ray Garrett Jr., former chairman of the Securities and Exchange Commission, described what the SEC considers to be the responsibility of the directors of publicly held companies as "a 'prudent or reasonable man' duty to investors to provide full and accurate information and otherwise to cause the company to comply with the federal securities law. It means adequate attention to the affairs of the company. It means adequate examination into the materials that the directors are asked to approve and authorize, and the relevant corporate procedures. Most of all, it means remembering that the director's duty is to investors and not to the individuals who make up management from time to time. It is our experience that the last of these most needs to be keep in mind."[7]

As the laws the hospital must comply with multiply, this would appear to be an apposite description of the duty of the hospital director or trustee, with the single exception that it is the community or the public, and not the investor qua investor, to whom the duty is owed. Joseph W. Barr, the former Secretary of the Treasury and director of several large corporations, who may be the business world's equivalent of the hospital's super trustee, told a conference of businessmen how he has performed his duties as a corporate director. When he became chairman of the audit committee of one board of directors, he related, he agreed with the management that he would "spend such time with the company as I needed to satisfy my own 'prudent-man' standards that the accounts of the company reflected as accurately as possible its true financial position. I estimated that this would take about 30 working days a year in addition to the meetings of the audit committee. I would not require a personal staff; rather, I would work through the various staffs reporting to the vice-president-finance of the corporation, and I would approach these staffs through the vice-president-finance."[8]

Describing how he spends the time he has for his audit committee chairmanship, Mr. Barr said: "I can engage in lengthy and detailed discussions with the staffs of the controller, treasurer, tax director, and auditor on the problems they are currently facing. The 30 days will also give me time for unhurried discussions with our outside auditors. These working sessions give me some added benefits that are impossible to quantify but are also difficult to gain from very occasional formal meetings. I get a chance to know and to evaluate the staff people in the financial, accounting, tax, and auditing staffs, as well as the people doing our outside audits. In addition, I think that I will, over time, get a feel for the business. I believe that knowing the people and developing a feel for the business builds up a better understanding of the numbers — especially in the debt management and revenue areas."

Because the business establishment in recent years has appeared to be under attacks from the public and the government, Mr. Barr was prompted to circulate his remarks about his "prudent-man" concept of directorship among his friends in the world of corporate finance, and he reported what they had to say. "The prompt and very thoughtful responses that I received indicated that I had touched on an important but delicate subject," he said. "Several respondents reacted very nervously to any implication that an outside director should be wandering around freely poking into all aspects of company policy. They were very apprehensive that such a procedure could stir up confusion and dissension and possibly a bit of politicking. My own experience leads me to agree completely, and I thought I had made the point: A director should function through the chairman or his designate and use corporate staff. The chief executive officer should know at all times what he is doing and to whom he is talking. Most respondents agreed that corporations have learned to live with audit committees, and any poking around in the company could best be done through this vehicle."

Mr. Barr represents a relatively new but growing phenomenon in corporate affairs: the professional director who serves on several boards and is well paid for his services. According to an opinion poll conducted and reported by *Trustee* magazine, only 5 percent of the hospital trustees surveyed were being paid for their services, although 28 percent reported that they received reimbursement for expenses incurred doing hospital business.[9] Twenty-one percent of those responding, however, thought trustees should be paid, giving as their reasons that the trustee who is really dedicated and involved spends a great deal of time at the job, and more and more time is required as the complexities multiply. "If trustees were paid, attendance would improve and turnover would decrease," said one. But others objected that payment would be incompatible with the concept of trusteeship of a not-for-profit institution. "If you are making a living and taking something out of your community, I feel that you should contribute some time putting something worthwhile back into it," said a Massachusetts trustee, speaking for the majority.

If hospitals are not yet far enough removed from their eleemosynary origins to comprehend paid professional trustees, certainly they are far enough into the era of public funding to justify a certain amount of organized, prudent-man poking around in financial affairs of the kind described by Mr. Barr, always with the proviso that this is being done with the knowledge and approval of the chief executive officer and through him or his designated representative. Especially, the need for experienced, objective financial judgment has grown in recent years as hospital capital accumulation has moved away from philanthropic gifts and government grants toward various forms of equity and debt financing. The shift has been dramatic. Fifteen years ago a hospital that borrowed money was looked upon as having somehow failed; there were a lot of them around, to be sure, but a mortgage was something you didn't talk about, like a cashier who embezzles. Today, in contrast, borrowing is involved to some extent in nearly all hospital capital expansion and is the major means of financing in most projects. Approximately half of all capital funds for hospital construction now are being furnished through borrowing.

Banks, investment houses, insurance companies, and other lenders have been quick to respond to a new and obviously promising market for their services, and a corps of hospital financing specialists has emerged to meet the demand. In fact, the sources and methods of borrowing have become so numerous that the need for specialists on the hospital side has grown correspondingly; vice-presidents of finance and comptrollers are in short supply, and administrators and trustees who are knowledgeable and sophisticated about money matters are an absolute necessity as each hospital has to consider which of the myriad options is best suited to its needs. The intricacies and questions relating to title, equity, interest, cost, conditions, terms, regulations, and legal implications all have to be sorted out; the financial feasibility consultant or adviser is as familiar a sight around the hospital as the chief of surgery, and the administration and board have to be just as much concerned about his competence and integrity. At a meeting of hospital executives not long ago, a financial consultant distributed a paper listing 96 questions or topics that had to be considered by the hospital contemplating a loan.

Since a large number of the most desirable of the financing options today are the tax-exempt revenue or general obligation bonds that may be issued by a political subdivision such as a city, county, district, or township under a transfer of title and leaseback arrangement, sound legal and political as well as financial advice is essential, and the knowledge and involvement of board members at every step in decision making are required. Only in their approval of staff credentials and quality assurance performance are trustees as obliged as they are here to observe Mr. Barr's prudent-man standard of "adequate examination into the materials that the directors are asked to approve and authorize."

Whatever the method of borrowing, financial feasibility depends ultimately on the hospital's own estimates of occupancies and revenues over the term of the loan. A banker whose institution has committed several hundred million dollars in hospital loans in the past four or five years told a group of hospital executives that once he was satisfied with the soundness of the occupancy projections and depreciation allowance and the acceptance of these, in addition to the interest rate, as allowable costs in the Medicare, Medicaid, and Blue Cross reimbursement contracts, as is commonly done today, he was usually ready to do business.

For most hospitals, a key provision of any long-term loan has been an open-end arrangement under which repayment of the principal sum may be accelerated as the hospital's own fund-raising efforts may permit. While it has been diminishing as a factor in the aggregate of hospital capital expansion, philanthropy is still providing in the neighborhood of 25 percent of all private hospital construction costs, and, in fact, the total of charitable contributions of all kinds rose from $12.6 billion in 1968 to $19.8 billion in 1974, about $1 billion of which was for health institutions and services.[10] Within the health services, the proportion of philanthropic contributions directed to hospital capital expansion has been diminishing.

"Within the nation's overall health activities, philanthropic agencies have tended to narrow their focus down to four points of concern," said Robert J. Blendon, Sc.D., of the Robert Wood Johnson Foundation of Princeton, NJ.[11] "The first is that private philanthropy has become a major source of first-stage, venture-capital support for the formulation of new projects or ideas. Philanthropic gifts tend to permit more flexibility during the critical embryonic phases of new activities [and] help to provide a legitimizing base for many health programs that go on to seek larger-scale public or private funding assistance. Secondly, philanthropic funds are often expended on projects that go beyond the limits of current governmental funding policies. Thirdly, private philanthropy often provides the 'critical glue' required to underwrite the losses of hospitals and clinics that serve low-income and poor patients without adequate governmental or private insurance coverage. Substantial numbers of people who are poor or near poor are not covered by existing governmental insurance programs, and therefore cannot pay for the full cost of the services that they need. By providing support for the substantial amounts of medical care rendered to these Americans, private philanthropy keeps many health institutions from bankruptcy. Although this philanthropic support is small in dollar amount, without it many of these health institutions could not remain solvent. Lastly, private philanthropy has become the key supporter of community-sponsored, out-of-hospital medical care programs. Today, 56 percent of all philanthropic personal health care dollars go for the payment of services outside hospital and nursing home care."

The evidence suggests that reliance on public funds for the support of health and medical affairs in the United States will continue to grow, Dr. Blendon concluded. "By the mid-1980s it seems likely that 50 percent of all national health expenditures will be derived from the public sector, with the bulk of the remaining funds coming from a heavily regulated private insurance industry," he said. "The growing sums spent by the public and private insurance sectors will continue to reduce the relative share of health expenditures provided by philanthropic giving. Consequently, private philanthropy must become much more selective in its choice of areas if it is to be effective. The need for private philanthropy to provide venture capital for new types of health activity will substantially increase. This need will be particularly true for out-of-hospital medical services and long-term care."

Views like these are not a cause for wild cheering in hospital board rooms. Trustees report that they are spending a measurable amount of their hospital time still on fund raising, as distinguished from other forms of capital financing, and professional fund-raisers say there is a reawakening interest in philanthropy on the part of hospital boards as it has become apparent in the past year or two that, contrary to what many had assumed up to that time, the government is never going to do everything for everybody. Describing the reasons for the changing atmosphere, William R. Haney, chairman of the board of Haney Associates, Inc., fund-raising counsel, said, "The eleemosynary dollar was needed to supplement or replace fickle federal funding, to provide necessary equity base for borrowings, and to decrease the size of high cost borrowings, because it was rapidly becoming the only remaining source of discretionary funds."[12]

Even philanthropic funds, however, are not likely to remain as discretionary as they used to be. Government economists and theorists, and some members of the Congress, are convinced that the tax laws should be revised to modify, and some say eliminate, charitable income tax deductions because the tax savings made possible for large donors determines the use to be made of large sums that would otherwise be available for public programs. As the proposition was stated by John H. Filer, chairman of the National Commission on Private Philanthropy and Public Needs, there is "concern at the ability of the relatively few to allocate so much of what is considered public, or at least publicly available, money."[13] Another view that has been expressed is that donors contributing support for facilities and services of hospitals participating in publicly funded programs like Medicare are in effect "creating an obligation for the commitment of public funds by private decision." If this is indeed contrary to public policy, as theorists have insisted, it won't last long as the certification-of-need requirements of the new planning laws begin to take effect, subjecting all facilities and services to prior public approval.

Moreover, there is a strong contrary view that philanthropy is one means of protecting the olive trees lovingly planted by previous generations, and that it should not be allowed to die in the era of public funding but should instead be vigorously defended and permitted to grow. Unquestionably, some tax reform measures and some form of national health insurance going beyond the public financing of hospital services ·that existed in 1975 will be enacted at some time during the last half of the decade, but it is the opinion of most hospital trustees that while these may modify the tax deductions available to wealthy donors in the past, and perhaps again narrow the focus of philanthropic interest in the health services, they will neither eliminate all encouragement for potential givers nor obviate the need for their gifts. It is likely, then, that trustees of the 1980s will be devoting at least as much of their attention to fund raising as they are doing today, and if it should be true, as Dr. Blendon has suggested, that the focus of interest for health service philanthropies at that time will be turned more toward out-of-hospital medical care, the interest of hospital trustees in sponsoring such services today suggests that the hospital will remain, as it has been in the past, the principal repository of such funds.

8. EVERYBODY CAN'T DO EVERYTHING

Ask a dozen hospital trustees what they consider to be the purpose or mission of the institutions they represent, and seven or eight of them will surely reply, "Why, to provide the best possible care, in the most economical way it can be done." Pursue the matter with a few more questions: What kind of care? For whom? Best in what way? Economical for whom? Now the answers are likely to reveal some unspoken, underlying assumptions: The hospital is expected to keep on doing what it has always done. The patients will be those referred by the doctors on the staff, plus those who walk in off the street, or fall in. Committees of the board and staff will satisfy themselves that the care is good. Of course, it costs a lot more than it used to, but doesn't everything?

A few of the others will have somewhat different answers, reflecting their understanding that the hospital has some new accountabilities relating to the things the institution does, not just the way it does the same old things. They know that the hospital mission now must comprehend community needs as these are defined by a group outside the hospital and that the measures of quality and economy also have some new dimensions. It's still our hospital, but now we have to prove that we're doing a good job and that the job we're doing is the job that needs to be done.

In any group of trustees there is going to be one, at least, who knows that it is really a lot more complicated than that. Not only is the hospital's mission defined and bounded by community planning, but the hospital's mission *includes* community planning—for all the health care needs for the whole population and the putative population for a generation to come. The capabilities that have to be measured against the needs are those of all the institutions. In this trustee's view, it is accepted as given that it is central to the mission of every institution to contribute what it can to the rationalization of the health care delivery system, so that both the system and the institution can survive. It is accepted also in this view that everybody can't do everything and that there must be some accommodation of autonomies among institutions.

This view has not been accepted easily anywhere, and there are places where it has not been accepted at all. "I can't see where we'd be any better off with five or six bigger hospitals than we are with twenty smaller ones," a trustee told a visitor who had suggested only that there might be some things some of the hospitals in his city could do together more efficiently than they could all do separately, as they had always done. "I suppose we'll have to come to it," another trustee in the same city said gloomily in response to the same suggestion, "but not yet." "This isn't the time" was a frequent reaction among trustees, and when they were asked why, the most common answer was "The doctors wouldn't stand for it." In most cases, as it turned out, the doctors had never been asked, though certainly there are many kinds of common enterprise or shared service that physicians would resist, as well as many that wouldn't affect them, or interest them, one way or the other.

On occasion, trustees who were queried about interhospital cooperation responded with a more substantial objection to this type of change than "this isn't the time" or "it wouldn't work." This was the misgiving that the sharing of medical facilities and services might be expected to diminish competition and thus impair excellence and somehow invade the American theological doctrine of free enterprise. Among trustees, physicians, administrators, and others who have examined and discussed this obstacle there are some who see it as a formidable barrier. But the more common feeling has been that it evaporates as one considers the essential differences between medicine and commerce. Many differences have been defined, in both law and practice, but the one that is at issue here is that the buyer or user of medical services, unlike the buyer of goods and services in commerce, commonly has neither the freedom nor the competence to choose the best value from among competing providers, and this is a circumstance that may make the buyer of medical services the victim of competition, and not its beneficiary as is commonly the case in commerce. When the competition among physicians is just for patients, and not for excellence, it may be the most flamboyant, or the most persuasive, or even the most unscrupulous, and not the most knowledgeable or skillful, who wins out, and when the competition among hospitals is just for patients and prestige, and not for the quality of service, the community and the economy may suffer rather than gain. It is argued also that the sharing or joining of services tends to diminish the kind of competition for patients and prestige that can be expensive, or even harmful, without affecting the competition for excellence that benefits patients and communities. Finally, if the coordination of services among institutions can result in a more rational and economical health care system, as the experience in some communities suggests, this result may act as a brake on the slide toward more and more government regulation, and it is probably unarguable that the American doctrine of free enterprise is at greater risk from the slide into regulation than it is from voluntary cooperation among voluntary health care institutions and services.

The fact of the matter is that cooperative action among health care institutions is not as voluntary as it used to be. The certification-of-need laws now in effect in about half the jurisdictions can make some degree of coordination mandatory. "The department is empowered to attach 'any reasonable condition' to its award of a certificate of need," said William J. Bicknell, M.D., commissioner of public health for Massachusetts.[1] "In early determinations the Public Health Council experimented with aggressive conditional certificates as an instrument to force rationalization of the health care system—e.g., requiring an applicant to negotiate an agreement with a neighboring facility on the consolidation of obstetric services before permitting him to renovate his own." Because in many instances such forcing actions turned out to be impractical, the Massachusetts department has limited its conditions of certification to those bearing directly on the applicant projects themselves, Dr. Bicknell reported. But the power to mandate change resides in the law in Massachusetts, as it does elsewhere, and as the National Health Planning and Resources Development Act of 1974 (Public Law 93-641) decrees that it shall do everywhere eventually.

With this prospect before them, trustees are changing their tune from "this isn't the time" to "the time is coming," and beginning to eye their institutional neighbors with interest and strike up exploratory conversations over the hospital back fences of the nation, feeling out the opportunities and the hazards of shared plans, programs, and services. There are models to be seen all over, ranging from simple, two-hospital communities where "you take the OB and we'll take the old folks" agreements have been reached in a few planning exchanges, to complex, multihospital consortiums that have evolved over years of painstaking planning and negotiating involving trustees, administrators, physicians, and community representatives.

One of the latter is worth examining, not as a plan that might ever be followed elsewhere but simply as a demonstration of the extent to which interinstitutional coordination can be carried when the conditions, and the people, make it possible. The seeds of the Detroit Medical Center Corporation were planted more than 20 years ago, when the Grace and Harper hospitals, side by side in an inner-city area, began meeting together, with no thought to do anything but share expansion plans, so that one should not leap ahead at the expense of the other. In time, this became an "improvement association," with other institutions also taking part, concerned with land use and acquisition in the downtown area. Later, the participating organizations formed a medical center citizens' committee that began to move from joint planning and development to consideration of shared services. In the 1960s, the group was successful in promoting urban renewal support for the creation of a medical center campus and began planning for the concentration of obstetric and pediatric services in two institutions. Then the Medical Center Corporation was organized with the explicit objectives of joint planning, coordination of services, avoidance of duplication of facilities and personnel, and concentration of specialized services in "centers of excellence."

For more than two years, committees representing the seven participating institutions in all the medical specialties met regularly, working through the problems to develop the plan that was accepted by the boards of the member institutions in 1973 and subsequently approved by the Detroit Area Planning Council. The plan calls for two of the hospitals to concentrate on general medicine and surgery and the principal medical and surgical specialties, with the exception of gynecology; another hospital will concentrate on obstetrics and gynecology; one will do only pediatrics; and one, only rehabilitation and long-term care. The Wayne State University Medical School, one of the member organizations, is to build a clinical facility where all nonemergency outpatient services will be provided for the area, and Detroit General Hospital, a city institution, will move to the medical center campus and handle all the emergencies.[2]

Many trustees and physicians recoil in horror when the Detroit plan is reported to them, objecting that it is too big, goes too far, will make referrals and consultations more rather than less difficult, and will result in further fragmentation and impersonalization of care—a criticism that is heard increasingly already at major medical centers. All these criticisms may be true to some extent; the Detroit planners have heard and considered them all and think their plan for implementation is flexible enough to avoid or minimize the difficulties. It may be, too, that the proximity of the institutions to one another and their long history of cooperative planning and action make possible a degree of integration that couldn't be accomplished anywhere else.

But it is plain that the new planning authorities are going to insist, at the minimum, that each institution's services henceforward shall be reviewed periodically in relation to comparable services at other institutions, so that there can be no repetition of the circumstance that permitted the development of six heart surgery centers in San Francisco a few years ago, at a time when the total volume of heart surgery for the area could have been accommodated comfortably in two. The result was that costs soared at all the centers. Moreover, it is believed that the many delicate skills demanded for a complex surgical procedure need to be in constant use to maintain the finely tuned coordination that is required. A surgical team that is idle may be one whose performance suffers.

In the past, these risks of expense and quality of hospital service have been private matters. If the trustees of Hospital A found that doctors and patients were choosing Hospital B because of, say, its superior radiographic equipment, they felt they had to go out and raise the $500,000 it would cost to get back in the race. The fact that there wouldn't be enough patients to keep both departments busy, if it was considered at all, wasn't seen as important. The charges would have to be raised accordingly, but the patients would pay. Or Blue Cross would. The one thing you can't do, the trustees all knew, is let a competitor get ahead, or stay ahead. Not in any business.

But this *isn't* any business. Not in the era of public funding. Half those bills today are being paid by Medicare and Medicaid, which are costing so much that the Congress and the responsible program executives are determined to do everything that can possibly be done to hold costs down, and this is the genesis of the new laws governing planning and use of hospital services.

Especially, the laws are aimed at cutting down any unnecessary expense at the core of the hospital—the bed. That there has been some overbuilding and overbedding in some parts of the country is now widely recognized. With Blue Cross and insurance paying most of the bills, nobody was too concerned when patients were admitted to hospitals as much for convenience as for necessary care. Hospital use was rising all the time with the growing population and the proliferating technology, and the beds were all needed, and the money was there. So if there were places where two new hospitals were both half empty, as happened sometimes, why worry? They would both fill up in time, and most of them did.

Some didn't, however, and when Medicare and Medicaid costs became a public problem and the Congress and the bureaucrats started looking around for somebody to blame, the empty beds lit up like neon signs. For a while, there was talk of a nationwide moratorium on hospital building, as though a surplus of beds in Orange County, California, could be relieved by forbidding construction in Boston, and some states and cities did impose freezes on hospital building for a time. Unquestionably, too, the publicity about surplus beds was partly responsible for the "industry out of control" concept that resulted in the harsh treatment accorded hospitals in the Economic Stabilization Program.

In planning, as in other aspects of regulation, hospitals suffered because the regulatory authorities in many cases were unfamiliar with the industry they were trying to regulate. The condition was described more than 100 years ago by John Stuart Mill in his celebrated essay on representative government. "I have known public men of more than ordinary natural capacity," he said, "who on their first introduction to a department of business new to them, have excited the mirth of their inferiors by the air with which they announced as a truth hitherto set at nought, and brought to light by themselves, something which was probably the first thought of everybody who ever looked at the subject, given up as soon as he had got on to a second."

So it was when at the White House, and the Department of Health, Education, and Welfare, and the Cost of Living Council, public men of more than ordinary natural capacity in a department of business new to them assumed that an empty bed anywhere was an unneeded bed and that therefore the difference between total bed capacity and total occupancy represented surplus, extravagance, waste. "Billion-dollar hospital bed overrun," said the headlines. Those who knew better demurred, pointing out that Miami's excess beds could scarcely have helped the pneumonia patients waiting for the chance to be admitted to one of Chicago's overcrowded hospitals, and that under any circumstances an occupancy of more than 90 percent of the total bed complement invaded the minimum safety zone required to accommodate emergencies, considering the obvious fact that beds are not interchangeable among hospital departments. An adult patient just won't fit into a pediatric bed, a circumstance that may have been overlooked by men of more than ordinary natural capacity bringing to light a truth hitherto set at nought in a department of business new to them. Commenting on the excitement, the American Hospital Association said that all these things, plus other uses for unneeded hospital beds, as for nursing home patients, had to be considered before any thought should be given to closing hospitals or units of hospitals, as some public men were suggesting.

While some of the cost and utilization regulations issuing from COLC and HEW may have reflected the "industry out of control" panic, the processes of developing legislation take longer, and there was time for everybody involved to get on to a second look in shaping the National Health Planning and Resources Development Act of 1974. As was mentioned in chapter 7, the act calls for establishment of a nationwide network of Health Systems Agencies having as their primary responsibility for their designated areas "the provision of effective health planning and the promotion and development of facilities, manpower, and

services to meet identified needs and reduce documented inefficiencies." The functions of the Health Systems Agency are:
1. Assemble and analyze data concerning the status of health delivery systems and resources.
2. Establish, review, and amend a health systems plan with health goals.
3. Establish, review, and amend an annual implementation plan with health objectives and priorities.
4. Develop and publish specific plans and projects for achieving the objectives established in the annual implementation plan.
5. Seek to implement its health systems and implementation plans with the assitance of individuals and public and private entities in its health service area.
6. Provide technical assistance to individuals and public and private entities to achieve programs in the health service plan.
7. Make grants and contracts to public and nonprofit entities to plan and develop programs and projects to achieve the health service plan.
8. Coordinate its activities with PSROs, model cities agencies, and other planning agencies.
9. Review and approve all federal grant money for health services.
10. Review and comment on needs for new institutional services.
11. Review appropriateness of all institutional services at least every five years and make recommendations to the state agency.
   (The initial review is to be completed within three years after the date of the agency's designation.)
12. Annually recommend to the state agency projects and priorities for modernization, construction, and conversion of medical facilities.

The Health Systems Agency may be a private nonprofit corporation, a public regional planning body, or a single unit of a general local government. The governing body, generally consisting of 10 to 30 members, must be nonproviders of health services. If the Health Systems Agency is a unit of a regional planning agency or general local government, the unit must have a specific governing body for the health planning function. All these activities are subject to review and approval by the state health planning and development agency, which is also responsible for integrating the area systems plans into a state plan—a task that seems certain to become sticky at the borders. Listed in the act as criteria to be considered when the area and state systems agencies are reviewing proposed changes in health facilities and services are, among others, the need for the proposed services; the relationship of the services to the existing health care system; the availability of resources; in the case of construction projects, the cost and methods of the proposed construction and the probable impact on costs of providing services; and the availability of alternative, less costly, or more effective methods of providing such services.

The provision mentioned in chapter 7 calling for the Secretary of HEW to establish a uniform system of accounting and reporting for institutional providers of health service and a uniform system for calculating rates has an added stipulation that seems simple enough on the face of it but promises endless complications. "Such system shall provide that rates reflect the true cost of providing services to each category of patient," this says, "and provide that differences in rates to various classes of purchasers be based on justified and documented differences in the costs of operation of health services institutions made possible by the actions of such purchasers."

Systems for determining cost by category of patient and rate by class of purchaser exist and are in use, but providers and purchasers don't always see eye to eye on the validity of the determinations. When the Medicare reimbursement rate was being negotiated, for example, the American Hospital Association insisted that patients over age 65 required more nursing service than the average patient and that therefore the nursing component of the Medicare cost allowance should be increased accordingly. To support its contention, the AHA conducted an intensive study of nursing services in a selected group of hospitals. The results were sufficiently persuasive, and eventually the Social Security Administration recognized the difference by allowing the inclusion of an 8.5 percent addition to the nursing cost component.

But in 1975 the SSA was under severe pressure from the Administration and the Congress to cut Medicare costs and, in retrospect, the results of the AHA study apparently became less conclusive; at any rate, the SSA proposed to discontinue the differential, and the negotiations started all over again. With 50 state agencies anointed under federal law to review costs and rates for all categories of patient and classes of purchaser, it is not comforting for hospital trustees to contemplate the opportunities for argument—not with the states holding the hole card that reads "Don't pay."

Of course, the law provides an appeal procedure, and a provider adversely affected by a decision of the state agency or the Secretary may always appeal to the courts for redress, and, as we have seen, the government doesn't win them all. But plainly the area and state systems are going to take their planning and rate review responsibilities seriously, and the hospital board that is not prepared to defend its cost data or has not itself carefully considered the "availability of alternative, less costly, or more effective methods of providing service," like a fighter who doesn't train for a bout with an opponent who has the advantage of weight and reach, is giving away more than it has to.

What are hospital boards of trustees doing now to prepare for Armageddon, if that is what is in store? All boards have planning committees, and most of these have plans, or master plans, and if they aren't up to here in blueprints at the moment, they are at least looking at the master plan from time to time to determine if the course of action foreseen at the time the plan was made still seems suitable. Some boards are going further and requiring their planning committees to examine all their assumptions in the light of new developments, considering that any plan needs to be looked at again and evaluated as far as possible in the way it would be seen by a Health Systems Agency.

"We took the position that any plan more than a year old had to be reviewed and any plan more than five years old had to be thrown out, and this led us into an intensive review and restatement of the hospital's mission," said a trustee whose hospital had moved into a wholly new building just a few years ago and thought at the time it was all set for a generation to come. "But look at what's been happening," he continued. "We hadn't figured on the surge in the demand for outpatient services and primary care, or the possible impact of utilization review on occupancy, or the certification-of-need laws. All the old questions had to be asked all over again. And then there were brand new questions, like what we should be doing about health maintenance organizations and one-day surgery —things that hadn't been heard of when we moved in here and thought we had it made."

HMOs have been around for years, though not by that name. Most trustees who pay any attention at all to what is going on outside their own hospitals know what an HMO is today, but not many have been looking at this development with a view to determining what its impact on their hospitals may be and what, if anything, the hospitals should be doing about it. The possible impact of freestanding surgery centers on hospital revenues is easier for trustees to see, once they are aware of it, but not all of them are. Some administrators and trustees have seen the surgical centers as a threat and hustled to make provision for same-day surgery at their own hospitals, seeking to forestall the initiation of freestanding units that would skim off some of the institutions' low-risk, high-pay business, and some have seen the same kind of threat in HMOs and have persuaded their medical staffs to organize prepaid group practices based at their hospitals. There may be good reasons against either kind of development at any particular hospital, but there doesn't seem to be any sensible reason a hospital shouldn't be taking a careful look at these phenomena. These may be available alternatives, or may at any time become available alternatives. The law says the Health Systems Agencies have to consider them in reviewing hospital plans, and the hospital that hasn't considered them first isn't going to look very smart.

Planning for health services in the fashion that is now envisioned in the law is not a new idea. As in the case of utilization review, the concept has been around for years, and there have been signals, for the most part ignored, that might have alerted trustees, administrators, and physicians that the regionalization concept now mandated in P.L. 93-641 was going to come. Regional links were proposed in the report of the Committee on the Costs of Medical Care in the 1930s, and again in the recommendations of the Commission on Hospital Care in the 1940s, and again in the Hill-Burton Act and the Comprehensive Health Planning and Regional Medical Program amendments that followed, and yet again in the report of the Secretary's Advisory Committee on Hospital Effectiveness. Published in 1968, this foreshadowed the planning provisions of the Social Security Amendments of 1972 (P. L. 92-603), as well as those of the later enactment. "However the planning function is staffed within the institution," said the Secretary's committee, "it is mandatory that the process must include the governing board, the administrator, appropriate members of the medical staff, and other personnel, such as nursing, representative of the services the institution offers. Especially, it is important for physicians to take part in formulating the institutional plan, not only because their patients and their responsibilities and their practices are central to the achievement of institutional goals but more particularly because medical staff and individual physician decisions and actions have a significant influence on every aspect of institutional effectiveness, from internal hospital management to developmental goals and interinstitutional plans for referrals and shared services. The physician who has taken part in the planning process may be expected to accept responsibility for the plan's effectiveness, and the one who has not, may not."

Planning agencies as their function was foreseen by the Secretary's committee were to be "as concerned with the organization and integration of programs and services as they are with the orderly provision of plant and equipment facilities. The most promising opportunities for advances in hospital effectiveness may be expected to result from the combined efforts of health care institutions, areawide planning agencies, and state authorities to encourage and when necessary demand the development of cooperative programs among institutions. The precise prescription of facility allocation and shared services in every case will depend on local needs and circumstances, obviously, but the committee is confident that when institutions and planning agencies are compelled to examine their facilities and services with a view to exploring every possible opportunity to achieve economies through integration, some such opportunities will be disclosed in every planning area, if not every health care institution."

The committee also said that prepaid group practice, now known and touted as HMOs, had "already demonstrated that health costs are reduced when physicians and patients are free of organizational or economic restraints on choice of institution and service, in the opinion of some authorities." This is still true, in the opinion of some authorities. For years, the Kaiser Foundation's comprehensive prepaid health plans and the group health cooperatives have been reporting substantially lower rates of hospital admission in their covered populations than are experienced in groups covered by Blue Cross-Blue Shield or insurance, because in these HMO plans all services are paid for and the participating physician has an incentive to keep patients out of hospitals unless they have to be there, whereas in Blue Cross-Blue Shield the incentive has been to get them into the hospital, where the return in paid-for services has generally been more liberal.

The cost experience has persuaded many professional health care authorities, most health theorists and economists, and practically all government officials and members of Congress that HMO is the way to go. But in spite of massive government encouragement in the form of loans and grants to groups interested in starting HMOs, growth has been much slower than anybody had expected, and the reason has finally emerged: Everybody likes HMOs except the two groups that are most directly concerned—doctors and patients. Doctors don't want to practice that way, preferring what they see, rightly or wrongly, as the more direct, personal relationship with their patients they have known in private practice. Patients like it better that way too, or at least they think they do.

Patients of doctors in the Kaiser, group health cooperative, and other HMO plans report as much satisfaction with their medical care as patients of physicians in private practice do, but when the HMO mode is explained to groups as an option alongside Blue Cross and Blue Shield, as it has been repeatedly in the past several years, the overwhelming response has been "No thanks." The pressure for HMOs will continue, because the appeal of the economy is real and persuasive. But the growth will continue to be slow, and any hospital board planning a commitment needs the advice not only of HMO enthusiasts but also of dispassionate experts.

While a few hospital boards are examining all these opportunities and options today, and all boards will be required to do so tomorrow, the preoccupation of planning committees still is with their own goals and plans, based on their own experience and their own view of their own communities. A man who has spent the greater part of his business life looking at hospital plans, and finding flaws in most of them, explained the process. "First, a hospital must look carefully at the composition of the population area it serves," said Harold E. Green, vice-president of American Health Facilities, Inc.[3] "Will the area change significantly? Will the makeup of its population change?" The answers to questions like these can usually be found in the offices of state and local health planning agencies, public health departments, city planning boards, or county commissions, and resourceful board members have often found the means for access to studies made by telephone companies and other public utilities, whose planning also begins with population movement.

"Then, a hospital must scrutinize its present services and their utilization, project changes in demand and in the way medical care is delivered, and ascertain what services should be provided in the future," said Mr. Green, describing in a few words a process that could easily occupy the full time of a planning committee assisted by a staff of experts for several months but must nevertheless be done as fully and as well as the individual hospital's resources will permit. "It must relate the size and makeup of its present medical staff to anticipated needs. It must project space requirements and the possible need for structural changes or additions. Relationships with other community health care providers also must be examined. What services do these other institutions provide? What are their utilization rates?" When all these factors have been carefully researched and evaluated, Mr. Green concluded, "the hospital can, with some degree of assurance, forecast long-range needs for facilities, services, and personnel. Unless a hospital carries out this study and evaluation process fully, it will have only a superficial, and not necessarily accurate, idea about what goals it should set for the next five, ten, or twenty years. A long-range plan is not a blueprint, nor is it a site plan showing where additions will be built or where new services will be incorporated. It is a narrative statement about a hospital's future, with some accompanying preliminary plans."

Obviously, to come close to developing and maintaining the kind of plan described by Mr. Green, the hospital needs not just a trustee committee that meets with the administrator once in a while to look at architects' renderings, as has been done in the past, but an active, interested, expert group of trustees with access to a planning staff. Depending on the size and resources of the hospital and its community, this might be either a full-time group of professional planners based at the hospital or a volunteer borrowed on occasion from the county commission, but the board isn't doing its job unless it is looking at all the questions and doing the best it can to find the answers with what it has to work with. "Build planning into operations" is the accepted prescription in corporations today, and the corporate executive who is a hospital trustee is beginning to bring the same demands he makes downtown into the hospital boardroom.

There's a long way to go. "Seldom is there recognition that alternatives to conventional, inpatient-oriented hospital construction projects may be preferable not only from the standpoint of costs but for accessibility and quality of care as well," said Dr. Bicknell, Massachusetts health commissioner, in his review of the state's certification-of-need experience. "This recognition is essential if better alternatives are to be developed, if the entrenched traditions of the hospital-based system are to be overcome, and if the potential of certification of need is to be realized." The planning mechanism by itself won't work, Dr. Bicknell explained, unless it is followed up by and coordinated with cognate licensure, financing, and utilization in an articulated regulatory policy. "There are many lessons to be learned from certification of need," he concluded, "but none perhaps so urgent as the importance of better coordination among separate but potentially complementary regulatory tools, both state and federal. Without that coordination, it will be impossible to test fairly the hypothesis that regulation can go beyond casting tomorrow's care in yesterday's mold, to serve the broadest possible consumer interest, promoting the provision of health care that is of good quality, efficiently produced, and accessible to all."

While it is likely that most hospital trustees, like most administrators and physicians, would consider that casting tomorrow's care in yesterday's mold is not such a bad idea, all of them understand that the trend of events is plainly in another direction. The coordination of regulatory tools may not seem the most desirable of all possible goals, but the regulatory tools are there, and they may hurt less if they are coordinated than they do now when they aren't.

Moreover, in spite of all the talk about alternatives to the hospital-based system, or the institution-oriented system, hospitals must necessarily remain at the core of whatever system is going to emerge, for a very simple reason: The hospitals have all the horses—land, plant, equipment, capital; professional, technical, and supporting personnel; organizational structure and management capability; and the vitally needed link to the community that exists in voluntary boards of trustees. No other elements of the health care system come close to the hospital in their range and depth of capability for delivering health services, and this is the reason so many analysts, including many of the public officials who have been the hospital's severest critics for so many years, consider that the hospital must be the focus of the regulatory effort. To expect that the health maintenance organization, or health care corporation,* or medical society foundation,* or freestanding surgical center, or any other newly created health construct could be developed separately from the hospital as the central organizational mode for the health care delivery system is to ignore reality, like thinking mom and pop could run General Motors. It isn't going to happen.

---

*See footnote on page 153.

9. WHY DON'T THEY WRITE ABOUT THE GOOD THINGS?

The late Ray E. Brown, a former president of the American Hospital Association who was considered by just about everybody to have been a leader of hospital thought and practice and by many to have been the best professional hospital administrator of his generation, once said that "public relations have been the architects of hospital operations in this country." It was his experience as a hospital administrator under several different boards of trustees, Mr. Brown said, that "We wanted nothing to happen to upset the community's image of the hospital. The last thing we wanted to get out to the community was a hassle either between the medical staff and the board or between different perspectives on the board. One reason a trustee doesn't always act aggressively is that he often values peace more than the broadening of service or the increasing of excellence. Until a few years ago, most of our capital was dependent on this image, so we couldn't risk a scene that might disturb our public appeal for funds."[1]

Before Ray Brown died, in 1974, the source of capital funding had shifted away from the public appeal for funds, and the emphasis in public relations had shifted away from projecting an image of peace. Nobody likes a public hassle any better now than he did then, but the trustee no longer gets to choose between peace and excellence. He chooses excellence, and the public relations effort is directed toward explaining what excellence is, and demonstrating that it's there and, if necessary, that it's more important than peace.

Like everything else the hospital does, the public relations task is a lot more complicated and difficult today than it was a few years ago, when the objectives were buttering up and loosening up the wealthy donors and making sure every-body knew about the wonderful work the doctors were doing, which everybody wanted to believe anyway. And did. Now the wealthy donors have been replaced by bankers, who want to look at the figures, and bureaucrats, who want to look at everything, and criticizing doctors and hospitals is not a sin against the culture, as it used to be, but a favorite indoor sport. The medical miracles that made the headlines a generation ago are accepted as a matter of course, and in fact demanded. It is the absence of miracles that makes headlines today.

Hospital trustees and administrators and physicians need to understand, as they sometimes do not, that these changes in values are not something that has been happening in the hospital world alone. Rather, they are characteristic of the whole society. As the population has become better educated, more affluent, and more mobile, it has also become more sophisticated and critical. Business, government, education—even the church—are all examined sharply and judged by their warts as well as their worth. Moreover, the processes of all our institu-tions, like those of medicine, have been technologized; as the doctor or nurse at the bedside has given way on occasion to the monitor and the oscillograph, so the professor has given way to the videotape, and the cashier to the computer. The resulting impersonalization of the social process has been less extensive in medicine than in other elements of society, but it is felt more keenly nevertheless, because the medical transaction is peculiarly personal, and the process is part of the outcome. Patients and their families may not always be aware of how much the process has been impersonalized, not only by the technology but by the multipli-cation of specialists and technicians diluting what was once a one-to-one personal relationship; when they are aware of it, they don't complain, for reasons that were made clear in the old Hindu proverb that said, "Before thou fordest the river, O Brother, revile not unduly the crocodile's mother!" But they feel the loss, nevertheless. When a sociologist investigator studying hospitals asked a patient what kind of day she was having, she beamed and replied, "A wonderful day—I got to talk to my doctor!"[2]

With this tendency for the miracles to be taken for granted and the flaws to be magnified, the hospital would have a hard enough time if its only public relations concerns were with patients and their families and the immediate community. And while these are still, as they have always been, the first circle of public interest that the institution is obliged to consider, the circles keep widening all the time, moving with the new accountabilities from the community to the area and the state and beyond. Obviously, the individual hospital is not directly responsible to the general public outside its own community; the accountability goes instead to the public surrogates in these widening circles: the representatives of consumers and purchasers and publics whose decisions increasingly determine how health care dollars are to be spent and thus have an impact on all hospitals. In turn, what the surrogates decide is determined by what all hospitals do and how well they explain and demonstrate their excellence. No institution is an island of itself; the empty beds in Miami could destroy the overcrowded hospitals in Chicago. More than most others, the public relations responsibility of hospital trustees is indivisible.

It is especially unfortunate, therefore, that the public relations responsibility is more likely than any other to be brushed off or ignored. Trustees understand and hold management strictly accountable for financial and operating results. They now understand and, albeit reluctantly, grapple with their responsibility for medical results. But they often appear unaware of any particular responsibility for how others think about their institutions, except as these opinions may relate to fund-raising results or, as Ray Brown suggested, a hassle that threatens the appearance of peace. Instead of setting goals and insisting that management make plans and submit budgets for public relations as it does for other programs, trustees are generally satisfied to see a budget line or two for public relations salaries and then grumble when a critical story about hospitals appears in the press. "Why don't they write about all the good things we do?" they ask the administrator. He doesn't know either.

Why don't they?

The first answer is that they do—a lot oftener than most hospital people realize or will acknowledge. It is hard to find a magazine or Sunday newspaper supplement that doesn't have an article about a new medical miracle promising hope for millions of sufferers, and a television freak who likes his miracles live in white coats can find them by twisting his dial at any time of the day or night. As a matter of fact, television entertainment and advertising glorifying doctors and hospitals were found by the President's Commission on Medical Malpractice to be responsible for a measurable fraction of the unrealistic public expectation that is at the roots of the malpractice problem.[3] The good things we do are also in the news every day. When the accident story on page one reports that the victims were taken to the hospital for treatment, and when the hospital's spokesman issues daily bulletins on the condition of the senator who is ill, and when the call goes out for blood donors who are urged to report to the hospital's blood bank—all these stories say, "The hospital is the place you need to be when you're in trouble." But let there be a lapse in the emergency department, as there always can be on occasion where human beings are at work under stress, or an unsupported charge of inefficiency by a politician seeking public favor, or a rise in rates, and let these be reported, as they will and should be, and the paper or the wire service or the TV reporter or the station manager is certain to hear the complaints: "Why don't you write about all the good things we do?"

The same sensitivity about the critical press is observable throughout the society. Universities, schools, businesses, churches, and public men and women whose names are news all have a tendency to forget the flood of information that reflects credit on their institutions and activities and remember only the drop of criticism. This phenomenon may have reached an all-time peak a few years ago when a vice-president proclaimed that the favorable impact of an hour-long lecture on television was wiped out by what was believed to be the critical elevation of a commentator's eyebrow.

Given all the disposition to forget what is good and remember what is bad, and all the sensitivity, there is still some substance to complaints by doctors and hospitals that the reporters who write about their affairs often seem to be "looking for trouble." There is also some substance to the complaint that when hospitals cooperate and tell reporters everything they want to know, and then some, as the Washington, DC, hospitals did in the celebrated case of the conflict-of-interest series in the *Washington Post* in 1972, the reporters more often than not will omit masses of explanatory detail and seize on whatever facts may be adduced to create a story of extravagance, conflict, scandal, or failure. This is seen as "reporting out of context," and it is the next most common complaint after "why don't they write about the good things?"

What is overlooked here is that everything that is reported is reported out of context except the verbatim recording of entire speeches or documents, and thus the question is not whether something has been reported out of context but whether the report has distorted the truth, and this is a matter of judgment. The reporter who has to write a five-paragraph news story about a five-hour meeting may have one judgment of what the truth is, and the chairman of the meeting quite another; the difference may be a matter of bias or distortion, as the chairman thinks, but it is much more likely to be a simple matter of judging what is news.

The essence of news is unusualness. This is the reason war and crime and riot and vandalism are news, while peace and lawfulness and order are not. This is the reason the medical miracle is news, and all the good things we do every day are not. This is the reason extravagance or conflict or scandal or failure in the management of public affairs is news, and good management is not. The way things have been going, there may come a time when good management in government will be so rare that it, and not bad management, will make news, and there may come a time when good management of quasi-public institutions like hospitals will be news for the same reason, but that seems unlikely. Meanwhile, bad management of public institutions will continue to be news, and reporters and editors will continue to consider that it is their job not just to report whatever bad management obtrudes but to investigate when there is any reason to suspect that it may exist, and then report what they find out.

It is a basic canon of the news business that the public has the right to know what goes on in public institutions. News people consider today that the hospital is a public institution, like city hall, and thus should be amenable to full investigation and disclosure. Most hospital trustees, administrators, and physicians acknowledge that the responsibility goes where the money comes from and some public "right to know" therefore exists, but they insist on protecting their rights of privacy also, and the law supports them where patients and physicians are concerned. A few trustees and physicians still regard the hospital as sacrosanct, and they would cling to the kingly doctrine that "We'll tell the peasants what we think it's good for them to know" as long as public policy permits, which will be only so long as they can survive without public funding.

There will be differences always between what hospital people see and what news people see as news and what they see as truth. It is a basic job of hospital public relations to comprehend both sides in order to minimize the abrasions that may result from the differences. This can be done only by the painstaking process of interpreting the responsibilities and tasks of each to the other, over and over again, and often under the pressure of time and circumstance. While these tasks can be performed for the most part by the public relations specialists on the hospital staff, there are frequent occasions when the administrator must be the principal interpreter, and, inevitably, there are times when trustees, too, become involved.

Whoever is answering the questions, the hospital needs an information policy as much as it needs policies governing admissions and contracts and unions. The trustees may decide that the policy should be full disclosure except where individual rights of privacy are involved, or it may be partial disclosure, with rights to know and needs to retain carefully defined, or it may be the closest thing the law and the sources of public funding will allow to kingly silence. But there needs to be a policy, known to trustees and physicians and administration and whoever may be or become the hospital's designated spokesmen, because nothing can upset the community's image of the hospital as much as answering questions one way Tuesday and another way Friday, or one way downstairs and another way upstairs. When this happens, it isn't the image of peace that is disturbed so much as it is the image of competence. The question that leaps to the mind of the inquirer is, "I wonder how they do in the operating rooms?"

As it concerns the news media, hospital information policy in many communities has been developed jointly by all the hospitals or by the local organization of hospitals, so there will be consistency of performance. It isn't easy to reach agreement on all the details, especially when some boards incline toward full disclosure and others toward kingly silence, but it has been accomplished in many places, and most successfully when not only the hospitals but the newspaper editors or reporters have been in on the discussions and helped to shape the policies. Where such hospital information practice codes have been developed, legal and medical advice also has been required. Policies governing the release of information in emergencies, particularly, have to comprehend the fine lines of privacy rights and the often tender sensibilities, as well as the rights of physicians in private practice and their local medical societies.

Hospitals having clear information policies established by the board don't always deal successfully with the news media, to be sure, but they are less likely than others are to fall into the obvious traps of inconsistency. Moreover, the administrator or public relations staff member or other hospital spokesman acting within known policy who is confronted with a question that can't be answered, such as one concerning the condition of a patient, can simply explain the reason for the policy instead of resorting to evasion, as is done so often, invariably arousing the suspicion of reporters.

In matters of finance, too, an evasive answer is always unfortunate. "What are they trying to hide?" is the instinctive reaction. When a hospital in the East was under investigation not long ago, for example, the administrator refused to disclose his salary; there was no policy requiring him either to disclose or withhold such information; he simply felt, understandably but unwisely, that it was nobody's business but his, and he wasn't about to tell. The reporter and his editor disagreed; they considered that a hospital accepting Medicare and Medicaid patients was spending public money, and the public had a right to know how. They made it their business to find out what the salary was, and in the process they discovered an expense account that wasn't anything out of the ordinary, actually, but did include some club bills that were disclosed along with the salary and made it look as though hospital executives were living in luxury on funds squeezed out of impoverished, sick old people. The salary itself was by no means excessive. If the administrator had reported what it was as soon as he was asked, it might never have been made public at all, or it would have been published and promptly forgotten. In any event, the absence of information policy made everybody look bad.

Policy doesn't relate only to information released to the press. What is to be said to employees? Physicians? Patients and their families? Visitors? Sometimes, information practice flows naturally from policies governing personnel, patient care, finance, and operations, but the manner of presentation and the detail to be included are not always clear. These are determinations for information policy. Increasingly, as a result of new public policy and consumer pressure, boards are leaning toward disclosure. Sooner or later it will be required of everybody, they feel, and hospitals might better come forth voluntarily instead of only under the lash of law and regulation.

As it relates to patient care, hospital information policy has been moving gradually out from under the traditional shroud of silence in which medicine was enfolded for so many years. Here the practice is changing not only in response to the general movement toward a more open society, but more particularly because of the growing recognition that information may be an element of treatment. In introducing its Patient's Bill of Rights in 1973, the American Hospital Association declared that "observance of these rights will contribute to more effective patient care and greater satisfaction for the patient, his physician, and the hospital organization." It was expected, the Association said further, that these rights "will be supported by the hospital on behalf of its patients, as an integral part of the healing process."

Eleven of the 12 specific patient's rights set forth in the AHA statement related wholly or partly to the information component of the hospitalization experience, the one exception being the underlying right to "considerate and respectful care," which is certainly not without substantive information content. Elsewhere in the bill of rights, information was referred to specifically. The patient, it said, has the right:

- To obtain from his physician complete current information concerning his diagnosis, treatment, and prognosis in terms he can reasonably be expected to understand, and to know by name the physician coordinating his care.
- To receive from his physician information necessary to give informed consent prior to the start of any procedure or treatment.
- To be informed of the medical consequence of refusing treatment.
- To grant permission to those not directly involved in his care to be present for case discussion, consultation, examination, and treatment, and to receive every consideration of his own privacy concerning his own medical care program.
- To expect that all communications and records pertaining to his care should be treated as confidential.
- To be transferred to another facility only after he has received complete

information and explanation concerning the needs for and alternatives to such transfer.

- To obtain information as to any relationship of his hospital to other health care and educational institutions insofar as his care is concerned, and to obtain information as to the existence of any relationships among individuals who are treating him.
- To be advised if the hospital proposes to engage in or perform human experimentation affecting his care or treatment.
- To know in advance what appointment times and physicians are available and where.
- To examine and receive an explanation of his bill regardless of the source of payment.
- To know what hospital rules and regulations apply to his conduct as a patient.

As a forthright departure from the traditional "papa knows best" attitude of the past, the Patient's Bill of Rights was newsworthy, and it was reported on page one of the New York Times. It had originated in the deliberations of an AHA citizens' advisory committee organized several years earlier in recognition of the growing influence of consumers in medical and hospital affairs, and most consumer organizations and public officials hailed the bill of rights as an enlightened move, although one, the Nader-affiliated Health Research Group, dismissed it as a public relations gimmick that wouldn't change anything.

In fact, though, it did. Some physicians protested that several of the enumerated rights involved matters physicians should decide and that adoption of the statement by a hospital would commit its physicians to practices they might not approve, and some hospital attorneys objected that a paragraph describing the patient's right "to expect that within its capacity a hospital must make reasonable response to the request of a patient for services" would invite abuses and possibly lawsuits. But some hospital boards adopted and publicized the bill of rights, or their own adaptations of it, and there haven't been any known instances of unreasonable or excessive demands for either information or services traceable to the new policy.

"A personal relationship between the physician and the patient is essential for the provision of proper medical care," said the introduction to the Patient's Bill of Rights. "The traditional physician-patient relationship takes on a new dimension when care is rendered within an organizational structure. Legal precedent has established that the institution itself also has a responsibility to the patient. It is in recognition of these factors that these rights are affirmed." Plainly, however, no hospital administrator in his right mind is going to insist on giving a patient information or service his physician considers inadvisable just because the AHA has said it is desirable. Association policy doesn't commit any hospital to doing anything it doesn't want to do. But the bill of rights has been accepted with interest and appreciation by patients and their families and representatives where it has been introduced. It has changed information practices in a few institutions; it has caused many to critically examine their information policies or the lack of any articulated policies; and the news reports of its adoption left the impression that hospitals understand patient care is something patients, not just hospitals and doctors, are concerned with—an impression that is sometimes unhappily and conspicuously absent from the hospitalization experience itself. One of the common complaints of hospital patients over the years has been, "Nobody will tell me what's going on." The Patient's Bill of Rights is a good start toward answering it.

Inevitably, the lack of a carefully thought-out information policy at the board level results many times in a corresponding lack of clear-cut public relations goals and programs. These can be furnished, of course, by an administrator who is himself interested and skilled in these aspects of his management responsibilities or by a talented public relations director or adviser. But more often the do-it-yourself administrator has considered that public relations begins and ends with his own public appearances and statements, and the public relations director, if there was one, was left to get out an annual report, publish a bulletin or newsletter or house organ of some kind for employees and volunteers, answer questions from reporters when the mayor's daughter had a baby, tabulate the responses to the patient opinion poll distributed every month, and furnish a convenient means of cutting the budget when a shortfall occurred in a really important department. All these activities, it was thought, would help build the kind of image the hospital wanted to have in the community and would answer the questions about costs that were assumed to be on everybody's mind, even though nobody ever really asked them.

In the era of public funding and consumer pressure, it is beginning to be understood that all these efforts need to be focused on specific goals, and then planned and programmed as carefully as nursing service or plant operations. For example, why does the hospital publish an annual report? Ask a trustee—any trustee—and he'll tell you it's done to "give the community an accounting of our stewardship," or some such vague, lofty purpose. Who gets it? Trustees, doctors, auxiliary members, volunteers, patients, donors, prospective donors, and "community leaders." But this isn't the community; it's the hospital itself, with the exception of only the donors and leaders, and nobody has thought to ask them whether they are interested in knowing anything about the hospital, much less everything. It is possible that hospital annual reports and house organs, some of them beautifully and expensively produced by talented people, may be the most widely neglected art form known to man. It is plain that not many trustees have been asking the kinds of questions about hospital public relations activities that they would ask in their own businesses: What are we doing this for? For whom? What do we want them to know? Why? How do we know they'll read it? Is there a better way it could be done? There may be places where all these questions have been asked, and answers have been sought for and found, and the activities continued unchanged. But the evidence suggests that there may be many more places where there are no real answers other than that it seemed to be a good idea, or everybody else was doing it. Hospital public relations budgets are not large, but it would appear that a lot of the money is being spent by hospitals telling themselves what they want other people to know, like giving temperance lectures to teetotalers.

The notable exception to this observation is seen in that part of the public relations effort that is directed toward fund raising, and the reason is simply that it *is* directed, or focused, on a specific audience for a specific purpose, and not just sprayed into the air with the expectation that the fallout may do some good with somebody somewhere. In contrast, the experienced fund raiser, or director of development, as they are now elegantly titled in hospitals and universities, is likely to know exactly what information he wants to get in the hands of what people to accomplish what objective, and he has a plan ready not only for the preparation and distribution of the information but for an organizational effort aimed at making certain the audience has got the message. If the hospital were to define the rest of its public relations objectives as precisely, make plans as carefully, and organize its follow-up effort as thoroughly as is commonly done in fund raising, some activities that are ineffective or, at best, unmeasurable might be discontinued, and some more productive programs undertaken in their place.

One of the new programs, surely, would be aimed at enlisting the physicians in the total hospital information effort. In their professional lives and activities, doctors and hospital administrators and trustees commonly and properly assume that the management of medical institutions and the medical care that is rendered within the institutions can be considered separately, as though they were discrete entities. Nobody else makes that distinction. To everybody on the outside, the doctor is as much a part of the institution as the walls and corridors, and a much more important part. To patients and families and visitors, in fact, and hence to the rest of the community, the doctor is the only visible link between the hospital experience and the rest of the world, the only component of the hospital that exists in the real world, and therefore the only source of information that is credible and reliable. The patient whose day was made joyous when she got to talk to her doctor was simply giving expression to what most patients feel, including those who never saw the doctor until they got there but who understand intuitively who it is around there who is really important.

So consider what happens in the typical experience: The patient, or spouse or parent or whoever, has a talk with the person in the admitting office who asks all the questions and records all the answers and hands out a little booklet that answers a lot of questions that haven't been asked but can't answer the only one that counts, "What's going to happen?" Then comes a parade of strangers on mysterious missions that remain for the most part unexplained. Somewhere in the procession of processions, if the patient is both blessed and lucky, there may be a glimpse or two, and a word or two, with the only person in the whole place who is both familiar and trusted, the doctor. At departure time there is another formal exchange in another little office with another stranger, who explains why the insurance didn't cover as much as everybody thought it would and hands out another little booklet telling why the rest of the charges have to be so high.

Eventually the patient is face to face again with the familiar and trusted friend, and when his anxieties are quieted he may ask about, or remark about, the costs—usually for the first time. In a minute or two, at that moment, either the doctor can provide the only information about hospital costs that is going to be both believed and remembered, or he can agree that the charges seem outrageously high and he can't understand them either, and completely destroy any credibility any other source of information about the hospital can ever have. There is probably no way any hospital can make certain all the doctors are answering all the questions just the way the hospital would like to have them answered, but unless the trustees and the administration have a systematic plan for keeping the doctors informed and stressing the importance of using every opportunity to inform patients and families and others, they are overlooking what is probably the most effective single method of creating and maintaining the kind of image of the hospital they would like the community to have. The thing that doctors tragically misunderstand is the importance of this information function *to them*; most of the regulatory constraints resulting from the "industry out of control" notion among government agencies hurt the doctors as much as the hospitals. Until physicians and hospitals can be brought to see themselves as others see them, that is, as one, the rest of the public relations effort is going to fall short of achieving its goal. There can be no public image of a hospital without the physician as its central focus.

In much the same way, though obviously with lesser impact, the hospital image is shaped by the behavior of other hospital employees, nurses first and most important, but all the others, too: the technicians and aides and therapists and maids and orderlies and admitting clerks and cashiers, not to mention interns and residents. How all these employees who see patients and their families are informed and instructed concerning their behavior is a matter that concerns management at all levels, in all departments.

But no matter how carefully plans are made and carried out, no matter how conscientiously the supervisors are instructing employees or how cleverly the personnel and public relations departments are in preparing their booklets and bulletins, the whole structure will fall flat if the employees really don't care. Attitude is everything, and attitude arises from sources that lie deeper than booklets and bulletins and meetings. Attitude is something trustees worry about. "The inherent problem the hospital has is getting middle management properly trained to train supervisors to get the people to know what's expected of them and how to do it," said a hospital trustee who is an officer of a bank. "Banks have the same problem. The turnover is tremendous among the teller and counter people who meet the public, and when you look for the causes you often find out they are dissatisfied because they haven't been adequately informed. They don't understand that the way they meet people, the way they say good morning, is part of the job, because that's never been explained to them. The same thing may be true, and it's a lot more important, in the hospital."

In a Chicago hospital, a new president who found what he considered to be evidence of low morale had a management consultant make a survey of employee attitudes that uncovered a lot of dissatisfaction with little things: parking space, inflexible work schedules, favoritism among supervisors—the kind of thing that can be found in almost any organization. But the consultant wasn't satisfied; the employees were acting more disgruntled than the reasons they gave could explain. So he probed deeper, interviewing more people, including some who had quit, and then he found the major cause: Nobody knew what was going on. The former president had barricaded himself in his office and communicated largely by means of memos, and, as often happens, this style of management in time had been duplicated all down the line. For example, the hospital had already purchased some property across the street and was planning to raze some old buildings to provide more employee parking space, but the employees hadn't been told about the plan. A whole new information policy was worked out and effected, and a visible improvement in employee attitudes soon became apparent. And a basic component of the new policy was that employees were to be assured, with repeated emphasis in demonstration sessions, that all their jobs included being polite and helpful in encounters with patients or visitors, because their behavior would help determine how well the hospital could do its job. Nobody had ever told them that before.

Obviously, saying it doesn't make it true. Unless trustees and administrators and physicians and nurses really think the emotional tone of the organization —the way its people behave toward one another and toward the institution's patients and visitors—is important to the result, nobody else is going to think so either. The orderly who sees a physician turn his back on a patient with a curt response isn't about to believe that the way *he* behaves matters to anybody. But it does make a difference. Experienced hospital observers like JCAH surveyors say they can tell within a very few minutes in a new place whether or not the people there really care about what they're doing. Asked how this can be so, they will say it is the behavior of the people themselves: how they look and move about, how they greet one another, how they address visitors and answer questions. "You can't measure it, but you can feel it," a consultant who has spent most of his professional life visiting hospitals likes to say.

Some trustees and administrators and physicians dismiss this as fantasy. Especially at the large teaching hospitals that represent the finest medicine practiced anywhere in the world, they argue, it is obviously ridiculous to consider that literally thousands of employees, many of whom belong to unions and are conditioned to think of the hospital more than anything else as an adversary, could be trained and motivated to make a favorable impression on patients and visitors, or that it would make any difference if they did.

One expert observer who disagrees with this view is Victor R. Fuchs, health economist and professor of community medicine at Stanford University Medical School, who said people who are troubled want to see someone, talk to someone, share their troubles with someone (see chapter 5). "As much as a cure," he said, "they want sympathy, reassurance, encouragement." They don't have to get it all from physicians.

Obviously, orderlies and aides and admitting clerks and cashiers aren't going to offer sympathy and encouragement to everybody who comes along, and so fulfill the caring function, but their behavior nevertheless contributes something to the quality of the environment that can be either reassuring or forbidding. It isn't all done by physicians and nurses. In fact, Dr. Fuchs questions whether the emphasis on scientific and technical medicine today sufficiently comprehends the caring role, or whether society could pay what it would cost if only physicians fulfilled it. One of his suggestions would look to the development of "multi-service organizations manned by volunteers and dedicated paraprofessionals expert in 'caring' by virtue of temperament and training. Such a service is probably most effective when provided by someone who cares by choice rather than by necessity."[4]

Most physicians do their best to see that the caring component is provided for their own patients, but under all the pressures of modern medical practice it isn't ever easy, and it is especially difficult in the confusion and complexity of hospital practice. Necessarily, the physician whose schedule requires him to become skilled at getting in and out of the room before the patient can remember what it was she wanted to ask him about has got to leave the caring function largely up to somebody else, and because the physician's behavior sets the pattern for everybody else in the hospital, that often means nobody is really caring.

Does it matter?

Some physicians think it matters a lot. One of these is Victor W. Sidel, M.D., chairman of the Department of Social Medicine at Montefiore Hospital and Albert Einstein College of Medicine, New York City. Dr. Sidel thinks concern for the whole patient, and in fact for the health of the whole community, should be included in any consideration of the quality of health care. He is disturbed because it isn't being done; if anything, concepts of quality are moving in the other direction. "When methods of determination of quality are devised largely by professionals," he said at a 1975 conference at the New York Academy of Medicine, "it is not surprising that they reflect the professional's view of the goals of the health care system. Since all too often professionals are the products of the intellectually oriented process which selected them and of the institutionally oriented, technology-centered process which educated them, it is no surprise that such professionals define quality for the most part in technical and professionally dominant terms. Most medical audit or peer review falls into this category."[5]

Because the technological components of care are relatively easy to measure and the social and emotional components extremely difficult, Dr. Sidel pointed out, quality assurance systems increasingly emphasize the former and omit the latter, and "hardest of all to measure and to relate to a specific form of care is its impact on the community." Yet the definition and measurement of quality will help determine how the resources are used, he said, "and will therefore determine which elements of health care will thrive and which will get relatively short shrift. If professionals bear the major responsibility for assessing the quality of health care and if they use the currently touted methods for determining that quality, the content, availability, and accessibility of care are likely to change, and, in my view, to change for the worse."

Dr. Sidel thinks the only answer in the long run will be to get nonprofessionals actively involved in quality assessment. This isn't going to be easy under any circumstances, he acknowledges, and it has elements of letting the passengers fly the airplane. But he is convinced that "part of the immediate professional responsibility for quality of health care is to educate and motivate community people to play an ever-increasing part in the process. In doing so the professionals will have to try to balance overall community needs against the needs of patients with specific problems. They will have to pay attention to patient and community education. They will have to respond to the academicians and specialists by asking: For whom and for what purpose does this represent excellence? Here as elsewhere the professional responsibility for health care is in my view to help those who receive the services take over the responsibility and the authority for the maintenance and the improvement of the quality of the care for their own health."

If this seems far afield from the public relations responsibility of hospital trustees, let them consider again what it is that they are trying to do. If it is, as has been suggested here, to explain what excellence in health care is, and to demonstrate excellence and by so doing improve the image of the hospital in the community and thus help to ensure the survival of the voluntary hospital system, then the first public relations responsibility has to be concerned with the people inside the hospital, because the image can never be anything more or less than the way the people behave. All the people.

10. SOMETIMES BECAUSE OF THE TEACHING HE HAS HAD

"Look at this garbage," the young physician said harshly. He flipped open the bulging file folder that lay on the table in front of him and started picking up pieces of paper—slips of all sizes and colors, sheafs of reports clipped together. "Just look at it," he said again. "Lab reports. Medication orders. Nurses' notes. X-ray. More lab reports. TPR. I've been through this once already. There are nearly 300 pieces of paper in here. No order. No organization. What good is it?" He glared down the table at the two dozen men and women seated there. Most of them looked at the note pads in front of them and fiddled with their pencils, but one or two glared back. They had listened attentively as the physician started to talk, but now they were getting fidgety.

These were members of the board of trustees and medical staff executive committee of a prestigious New England hospital. They had come up here out of season to a famous seaside resort to spend a day and a half talking about the hospital's problems and its future course, and here was this young doctor, a stranger to most of them, haranguing about somebody's badly organized medical record. What did it have to do with them? What was the point? Let's get this over with and get on with what we came here to discuss. What was he saying now?

"Could anybody look at this goulash and get any clear idea of what was going on?" is what he was saying. "Could anybody remember enough of it to make sense out of it? Could you?" He glared down the table again, challenging.

One of the doctors wasn't taking any more of this. "Possibly not," he said, "but you'd remember the important things, and anyway that's obviously not the kind of record you'd find in any well-organized hospital." He glared back.

The young physician disappeared from view, bending over and reaching under the table. When he stood up again he had an armload of file folders that he started piling up on the table in front of him, all bulky, some with papers spilling out. They all looked like the one he had been talking about. He looked up and grinned.

"Ladies and gentlemen," he said. "These folders all came from your own medical record library. I picked them up yesterday afternoon on my way up here, with the permission of Larry," he nodded at the administrator, sitting beside him at the end of the table, "who agreed to help me make a point. It is simply that the practice of medicine has become so complex—so many facts, so many possibilities to consider, so many theories to test and rule out—that it simply isn't possible, in any but the simplest cases, to *remember* everything that has to be remembered even for a single patient, much less for the half dozen or more each of you may have in the hospital at any one time. That's why we have records, of course. But records like these aren't as much help as they could be. It's too easy to overlook something in these masses of unorganized detail. At best, you spend more time than you can afford to, just looking for some fact you need to know and know you've forgotten."

One of the doctors interposed. "Are you suggesting that it's all going to be done by computers?" he wanted to know.

"Eventually, yes," the young physician replied. "But not necessarily for all of you, and not right away for any of you. Of course, the records I picked out to bring to this meeting are obviously bad examples. But they *are* your own records, and they illustrate the problem that exists for all records—all practice—to some extent: the need to organize a data base for every patient that will ensure against overlooking some significant detail."

Not all the doctors agreed. The records committee may have missed some derelictions that needed correction, it was acknowledged. This was embarrassing, but it was scarcely a cause for changing the whole system. But as the discussion moved along to examine some of the new demands for quality assurance, it was emphasized repeatedly that quality has to be *demonstrated*, and records are essential for demonstration. "The JCAH has been saying for years that good records are not just *evidence* of good practice, but *part* of it," the young physician said, "and now the laws and the regulations and the courts are saying the same thing, and the new data systems are making it possible for them to find out how good you are—and easy for you to show them."

The mention of courts got everybody into the act. One of the older physicians in the group was certain that the PSRO data systems were going to increase malpractice liability, not diminish it. "Some norm will be established in Ohio for a procedure we stopped using years ago here in Connecticut," he predicted, "and we'll have to go to court to prove that it isn't any good." But JCAH lawyers and physicians had made a study of the laws and court decisions relating to utilization review and malpractice and concluded such fears are almost wholly unfounded, somebody else reported.

As this part of the day's program ended, the chairman of the board of trustees reminded the group that the purpose of the meeting was not to take formal action on anything, but to examine the hospital's problems and purposes. But he asked the chief of the medical staff to make a report on utilization review, in the light of the discussion here, at the next board meeting.

During a break later in the day, one of the trustees was talking to a reporter who had been invited to attend the meeting as an observer. "I didn't understand all of it," the trustee said, referring to the discussion of medical records and utilization review. "But I understood a lot more of it than I thought I was going to when that young fellow started to talk, and for the first time now I'm convinced that this board can do something about patient care besides listening to the doctors' reports that everything is all right, and that we damn well *better* do it."

Board-staff-administration seminars, or retreats, as they are often called, are an increasingly popular method of conducting educational sessions for the responsible leaders of all three groups. Like the one reported here, these meetings usually are conducted with the assistance of outside speakers or consultants who bring a new perspective to the hospital's problems and activities and, as the young physician did, initiate discussions that go beyond the immediate interests of the participants to the general concerns of the health care system. A hospital consultant who has arranged and taken part in a number of seminars of this type considers that the most valuable contribution the program can make arises from the discussions following presentations by outsiders on such subjects as planning, finance, utilization review, HMOs, and national health insurance. He explained why: "In every discussion, there are going to be varying views within the group about what the speaker has said, what is the significance of the trend or movement or activity he has described, what it means to the hospital, and what the hospital's policy or response should be. But when the focus of the discussion is outside, not inside, the hospital itself, these varying points of view are apt to be presented more dispassionately, and the disagreements—there always are some—tend to be less abrasive. One of the main purposes of these meetings is to develop the hospital's esprit, the feeling that we are, after all, engaged in a common enterprise, and we have to understand and help one another. Arguments that illuminate the various points of view contribute to this feeling, but heated disagreements don't, so it is wise to shift the focus outside our own activities, at least some of the time. They get back there pretty quickly anyway. But our clients have found these meetings to be great morale boosters."

To help foster the feeling of objectivity and removal from the immediate pressures of hospital routine, the consultant favors the retreat aspects of the seminars he plans for his client hospitals and insists that they must be held away from the hospital and, if possible, in the relaxed atmosphere of a resort environment offering some opportunity, and some time, for recreation. He considers that these apparently irrelevant factors make an important contribution to the team spirit that is one of the goals of the conference, and that in fact the environment and emotional tone of the occasion contribute to the learning purpose. "Corporations found this out long ago," he said. "You can bet that the reason so many sales meetings and management conferences and executive training sessions are held at Freeport and Bermuda and Point Clear isn't just that the corporations can afford it and the managers like to have a good time. The chief reason, without any question, is that they get better results. If it works for business, why not for hospitals?"

There are two reasons why not, in the opinion of some hospital people. One is that the cost squeeze makes it necessary for hospitals to save on expense in every possible way, and educational meetings away from the hospital would appear to be an unneeded expense, even if many of the participants are willing to pay their own way, as many do. The other reason is that some consider the nature of the hospital mission, the not-for-profit character of the organization, and the fact that most hospitals ask for and receive contributions for the support of patient care make it inappropriate for hospital business to be conducted on the same level as that of wealthy corporations. Besides, it is argued, it isn't necessary. The content of the meeting and the conduct of the participants come from the people themselves, not the surroundings. With the right kind of planning and preparation by the administrator and his staff and whatever consultants or others outside the hospital organization he may want to call on to help, constructive and productive seminars can be held in the hospital's own boardroom, auditorium, or cafeteria. Inevitably, there will be interruptions, but these can be minimized and needn't be damaging to the purpose of the conferences.

"Our board formed its own committee to decide what a proper trustee education program should be," said Lad F. Grapski, president of Allegheny General Hospital, Pittsburgh.[1] "About once a year, the trustees, principal administrative officers, and principal physicians meet for a seminar which is usually held from 10 a.m. to 3 p.m. on one day. These are always well attended, because they are sponsored by the trustees themselves. They have decided what they want to hear, and they are ready to listen to it. One year, for example, they decided to work with our state legislators. They developed a legislative seminar. The trustees; the physicians, and the administrators invited the local legislators to come in and learn what our problems are, then talk about how we can work together most effectively. We all learned something that day. Usually, however, these programs have to do with management—that is, clinical management, administrative management, nursing management, any kind of management the board has to be concerned about. Recognition of the issues and considerations of the various alternative methods of dealing with change and making decisions are what we are involved in.

Another hospital that developed its own educational program to meet its own needs is the 95-bed Memorial Hospital in the small community of Watertown, Wisconsin, where the initiative came when administrator Leo Bargielski decided that there is too much responsibility today for one person to make all the decisions without the opinions and advice of board members. The board members, he suspected, needed to be better informed about the hospital's operations and the health care system generally in order to take their part in decisions. Particularly, he considered, the most important areas of concern were with the legal status and corporate responsibility of the hospital, the relationship of the board and administration, and the role and relationship of the board and the medical staff. To find out how members of the 15-member board viewed these matters, he undertook a questionnaire survey as a base for determining their information needs. "They knew a whole lot less than I thought they did," he said, commenting on the result. "I think if any administrator undertook a similar survey of his board members he would find a lot of things that would startle him. Administrators think they are keeping their boards up to date, but a survey would probably disclose a lack of understanding of governance fundamentals."[2]

To bridge the information gap, Mr. Bargielski designed a nine-hour curriculum consisting of three three-hour class sessions dealing with hospital-community affairs, board-administration relationships and hospital operations, and board-medical staff relationships. The board was divided into three groups that came to the hospital for the three-hour afternoon classes over a period of three weeks. Faculty members included Mr. Bargielski, the hospital controller, the chief of the medical staff, the director of nursing service, and the hospital's legal counsel. For each phase of the program Mr. Bargielski developed a reading list, and trustees were furnished copies and given assignments to prepare for the lecture and discussion sessions. Only one board member failed to show up for the classes, Mr. Bargielski reported, and "class discussions were lively. Many, many questions were asked. The Tapes for Trustees furnished by the Hospital Research and Educational Trust were used as teaching aids, played during the sessions, and proved helpful in stimulating discussion."

Now Mr. Bargielski has developed a condensed version of the course as an orientation program for new trustees, and a continuing education program to keep board members up to date. "The orientation program teaches trustees that a board member has a commitment to both continuing education and active participation in board meetings," he said. "We now have an annual evaluation of board members based on attendance and participation. If members are not participating, they are asked to change their ways or leave." Another result of the program has been a thorough revision of the bylaws of the hospital and the medical staff. "The board went through the articles of incorporation and the bylaws line by line to be sure that the modernized version would reflect recent court decisions and JCAH requirements," Mr. Bargielski said. "My title was changed to executive director, and I became a member of the board. This action makes the relationship between the administrator and the medical staff much clearer, because I now represent the board in my role at the hospital. One of the major achievements of the education program is the board's current understanding of the need for medical staff account-ability for the medical care provided in the hospital. As a board member, I no longer have to act as a messenger for the medical staff, interpreting medical matters to the board. The chief of the medical staff is now on the board meeting agenda and reports directly to the board, and thus to me."

In the continuing education programs, Mr. Bargielski has started to bring in outside speakers. One panel discussion featured executives from the state hospital association and state medical society and the chairman of the board of trustees of a large urban hospital. "Our trustees really paid close attention to what the board chairman on the panel had to say," he reported. "This gave me a message that for future programs it would be a good idea to bring in board members from other hospitals as speakers. Most trustees, not being health care professionals, relate best to what their fellow board members say."

Not all hospital trustees are that avid for learning, however, and not all administrators are committed to trustee education programs. "Most of my board members are executives or directors of huge corporations or financial institu-tions," said the administrator of a well-known midwestern hospital, "and they just can't believe the management of a $50 million business can be all that compli-cated. They look at the reports, and ask a few questions, and leave the details for me to handle." An Ohio administrator had a similar report. "I sent the board members some of the material that's been coming out on utilization review," he related, "and at the next meeting it was plain they hadn't really looked at it. One of them said, 'You take care of it. That's what we pay you for.' "

A few years ago, that was the way most administrators wanted it. But Medicare and Medicaid, utilization review, the new planning laws and regulations, and perhaps most of all *Darling* and *Nork*, have left so many notches where the limb can be sawed off that not many administrators want to be out there on the end of it all by themselves. At the very minimum, they want trustees to know enoiugh to play a constructive reacting role in the management of the institution. This role was described not long ago by Robert K. Greenleaf, a retired corporation executive who has been a trustee of a number of institutions and foundations and has written extensively on the subject of trusteeship. "In the reacting role," he said, "trustees usually do not initiate or shape the character of the institution, nor do they see it as their role to examine the traditional wisdom. If they are conscientious, and most of them are, they will do the following: try to install competent operating officers, support and encourage them, maintain some gross controls by requiring trustee approval on certain major actions, check such data as they have for evidences of serious malfeasance, and affirm, deny, or modify policy questions that are submitted to them."[3]

But most administrators today consider that this reacting role is no longer good enough for hospital trustees, given the new forces institutions have to contend with. Mr. Greenleaf agrees. What is required now is to put trustees into an affirmative role, he said. "They should proceed to design a new role for themselves, and be prepared to invest the time required." The principal dimensions of the new role, as he then explained them, are:

- *Setting the goals.* What business are we in and what are we trying to accomplish in it? Profit-making business firms have some trouble with this question. Other institutions have a great deal of trouble with it. The first thing an institution needs to do in order to start on a conspicuously higher course is to state clearly where it wants to go, whom it wants to serve, and how it expects those served directly, as well as society at large, to benefit from the service. Unless these are clearly understood, an institution cannot approach its optimum performance. Yet the internal administrators, left to themselves, usually hesitate to state goals so precisely.
- *Performance review.* Since the administration is involved in the performance of the institution, part of the data which trustees use for their overseeing role should come from a source that is independent of administration.

- *Executive growth and selection.* Every large institution that is to be optimal in its performance must produce leadership out of its own ranks. It should import some leaders and other trained persons in order to check inbredness and keep the organization stimulated. Growing people, bringing able people from other experiences, should be a constant concern. However, some otherwise able administrators become so preoccupied with day-to-day performance that they sometimes neglect this vital organization-building work that needs constant attention. Therefore, close overseeing of executive growth and selection is suggested as an explicit function for trustees.
- *Organization of the top executive office.* The organization of the top administrative office and the assignment of functions are not things that the members of that office can do well. They can do them for other parts of the institution, but not for themselves. Left to themselves, they work it out somehow, but optimal institutional performance does not result. Because they are not administrators and therefore do not have this problem, trustees are in a position to have the objectivity and perspective on the institution to work this out.
- *Maintaining openness to change.* Occasionally an inside administrator will detect, in time, the need for a new pattern and effect a change in course, but the structure does not favor it. Sometimes when the administrator does detect the need for a new pattern, he is unable to move the institution. Just keeping it operating on the old pattern presses his leadership to the limit. In such a case the risk of change looms as a greater threat than the risk of failure. The critical signals are those that tell one that action should be taken today in order to forestall impending trouble tomorrow. These are the signals calling for change *now* that the busy administrator may miss. The trustee has a better chance than the administrator to be open to change. In fact, this is his or her role—to maintain openness to change, which his or her relative immunity from day-to-day operational pressures makes possible. Yet administrator and trustee are not sharply differentiated roles. In fact, they are a close mesh, in which the administrator should be mostly dogma and a little bit open to change, and the trustee should be a little bit dogma and mostly open to change. The two roles, closely linked and working in harmony, should take care of both today and tomorrow.

For either the reactive or the affirmative role, or whatever combination or variation of them the board may have seen and chosen as its proper response to the new demands on the hospital, board members need more information than they have commonly had in the past, and they know it. Orientation and education programs for trustees like the Connecticut hospital's elegant retreat and the homegrown kinds at Pittsburgh and Watertown are being developed all over. In many communities, hospitals have joined forces in joint trustee programs; state and regional associations are sponsoring trustee conferences. Institutes and workshops abound. Manuals multiply. Yet in its 1974 survey of trustee activity the American Hospital Association found that nearly 40 percent of the respondents hadn't attended a single meeting of a local, state, or national health care organization for over a year, and 45 percent said their hospitals didn't have any systematic program of orientation for newly elected trustees.[4]

In his study of the governance of teaching hospitals in New York City, Russell Nelson, M.D., discovered that "in most institutions, both the orientation and continuing education programs are informal to the point of being haphazard. Typically, the new trustee early in his term of office will spend an afternoon at the hospital talking to the administrator and perhaps the chief of staff, the director of nursing service, and one or two department heads, most of these interviews occurring during a fast tour of the premises. From that point on, it is assumed that the trustee will inform himself by reading such reports as are made available to him, possibly including a subscription to one or another of the relevant publications, and by attending meetings of the board or of a committee to which he may be assigned. On occasion, he may be invited or urged to attend a hospital council meeting or seminar conducted by a hospital association for trustees, administrators, and medical staff members, where he may hear something that he can apply in one way or another to his own trusteeship, but where more often than not the presentations are so general that they have little real value for him."[5]

In an extensive study of hospital continuing education completed in 1974, Daniel S. Schechter of the American Hospital Association also found more failures than successes.[6] "Workshops, seminars, institutes, and convention programs planned for trustees have often been poorly attended," he reported. "Some trustees, explaining that they have little time for attending meetings, suggest that an administrator attend the meetings and summarize the proceedings for the board, while others complain that institute faculties are usually dominated by administrators. Many support the idea of one-day local workshops and local informational sessions with members of the staffs of state hospital associations, who might travel through the state to meet with hospital trustees. State hospital associations that have planned educational workshops have had uneven results. It may be significant that one association attributes its success to the continued involvement of governing board members in designing programs planned for them, while another association, distressed by the small attendance at its trustee workshops, acknowledges that one reason might have been the fact that administrators and association personnel planned the programs for trustees, 'who wouldn't know what issues it was important for them to understand.' "

One authority has suggested that the difficulty may lie not so much in the information techniques or instructional methods as in the lack of motivation for learning that has prevailed in the past. "The traditional role of the hospital board, in which the board merely receives monthly or quarterly reports on past perfor- mance, frustrates both the interest and the potential contribution of the trustees," said Nathan Stark, a long-time corporation executive and hospital trustee who has now professionalized his interest and is vice-president for health affairs of the University of Pittsburgh.[7] Mr. Stark believes that changing the organization to give trustees active roles will motivate them to be able to deal effectively with the issues. "As an example, he suggests forming temporary task forces of trustees and qualified professionals, with assistance by the administration, to work on particu- lar problems, such as those that require adaptation to changing environment, collaboration among many groups or agencies, or intense commitment to the hospital's goals. He believes that the trustee's skills in problem solving could be put to work in this kind of organization to deal with such matters as outreach programs, neighborhood clinics, home health care, ambulatory care, medical education, and relationships with other health care institutions and agencies," Mr. Schechter reported.

It may be that the active involvement in hospital affairs that is needed to spark the desire to learn is coming whether boards plan it that way or not, because all the new accountabilities that have been described here will demand it. If that is the case, the need is simply for carefully planned, well-organized information pro- grams, with more emphasis on the content than on the manner or circumstances of presentation. The minimum information needs, according to Mr. Schechter, are those relating to:

1. Legal responsibilities of the board
2. Management policies of the hospital
3. Relationships between the hospital and physicians
4. Social and economic factors underlying changes in health care delivery and financing
5. Community planning for the allocation of health care
6. Current and proposed legislation affecting the delivery and financing of health care

"In addition to this general knowledge, trustees need specific information about their own hospital in order to make policy decisions—the kind of informa- tion that will help them to pose questions regarding the allocation of resources (for new services, for example) or alternative courses of action," Mr. Schechter said.

"A basic requirement is accurate financial data, interpreted by the administrator. Trustees also need sufficient information on the utilization and costs of the various services, and on the expressed needs of the patients and the community, to judge whether the hospital's services are accessible to those who need them and at the least possible cost. At the same time, the board must hold the medical staff responsible for demonstrating that it is maintaining and improving the quality of medical care."

Where motivation exists, information is never far behind. The trustee who wants to learn will have a harder time avoiding information than finding it. His own hospital is certain to have an office or library full of trustee reading material, and probably tapes and films as well. The regional and state hospital associations all publish information prepared especially for trustees; their newsletters and bulletins are informative and reliable; some have trustee manuals that member institutions use for orientation of new trustees. One of the most complete and informative of these ‧is *Health Care Governance,* published by the Tennessee Hospital Association, a compilation of materials with basic information covering every phase of hospital operations and a condensed chapter on current trends in health care delivery. For the trustee whose interest knows no bounds, the AHA has, in addition to its monthly magazine *Trustee,* a current publication including a selection of the most topical and relevant of the articles published in that journal over the past several years, and the AHA also has a long list of readings and instructional materials for trustees. Even the United States Chamber of Commerce has a publication, *A Primer for Hospital Trustees,* with a bibliography of more than a hundred books and articles recommended for the eager learner. "Of making many books there is no end," said the preacher in Ecclesiastes, "and much study is a weariness of the flesh."

Because there is so much material available that no trustee can possibly encompass and evaluate it all, selectivity is essential, and so the few must choose for the many; ideally, each board will organize the learning program for itself, obviously with the assistance of the professional and administrative staffs.

Dr. Nelson described how the process might work:

"It is recommended that the hospitals should initiate comprehensive, systematic information programs for their present board members aimed at making certain that all of them have the opportunity to become familiar with the business, professional, and public operations of their institutions, including current programs and problems and future plans for development. This training could include 'state of the nation' reports by heads of all the principal departments, with time for questions and discussion, and presentations by representatives of the medical services, including appropriate examination of failures as well as triumphs. Following this kind of basic training, which could readily be adapted as an orientation program for newly appointed trustees, and might also be conducted jointly for groups of trustees representing several hospitals with similar structures and functions, the continuing information agenda for trustees should be directed toward keeping them up to date on events and developments elsewhere in the health service system. Here the method might well be to introduce a series of lectures or discussions dealing with city, state, and federal regulatory and financial responsibilities; reports by medical educators on house staff training; the new emphasis on primary care; and other matters certain to have an impact on teaching hospitals over the years and therefore very much the concern of teaching hospital trustees. Other experts could be called on for discussions of health maintenance organizations, professional standards review organizations, national health insurance, the new planning legislation, and the trend toward hospital consortia, satellites, shared services, joint ventures, and multiple unit management systems—again, all movements with which hospital trustees should be prepared to deal in the future."

But as Jacques Barzun of Columbia University, one of the great teachers of our time, said again and again in his essays and lectures, education is intangible and unpredictable, its result depending as much on the student as on the teacher. "Education comes from within," he wrote; "it is a man's own doing, or rather it happens to him—sometimes because of the teaching he has had, sometimes in spite of it."[8] William James explained how the educated mind responds: "Just as our extensor muscles act most firmly when a simultaneous contraction of the flexors guides and steadies them, so the mind of him whose fields of consciousness are complex, and who, with the reasons for the action, sees the reasons against it, and yet, instead of being palsied, acts in the way that takes the whole field into consideration—so, I say, is such a mind the ideal sort of mind that we should seek to reproduce in our pupils."[9] In the complex years ahead, the hospital will be fortunate whose trustees see the reasons for and the reasons against and, instead of being palsied, act in consideration of the whole.

11. SOME WILL BE MOVERS AND MANAGERS, SOME WILL BE MOVED AND MANAGED

In an essay that revealed his fascination with the future, the French philosopher Pierre Teilhard de Chardin wrote that "Like nervous passengers in a ship or an aircraft who turn their eyes away from the ever-moving emptiness of sea or air, we generally shun the prospect of the future into which we are launched. Clinging to the apparently more solid framework of the past, we try to forget the bewildering domain of possibilities in which we are swallowed up." Chardin would have been astonished at the extent to which in a few short years the passengers have got over their nervousness and are now straining their eyes at the emptiness looking for the possibilities and even trying to measure them with their computers. This is not to say, however, that the passengers are not still clinging to the solid framework of the past.

Thus, when a group of eminent and learned passengers known as the Club of Rome recently put all the possibilities they had glimpsed into a computer at the Massachusetts Institute of Technology, which then estimated that the planet would run itself out of food, fuel, and space within a few years unless its basic values and directions were changed,[1] other passengers, equally eminent and learned but with a stronger grip on the framework of the past, cried out that their glimpses of the possibilities hadn't been considered, or considered enough, by the

Club of Rome computer, and no such changes of values and directions were needed at all.[2]

The same diversity of possibilities and modes of thought about the future results when the passengers strain their eyes only at that part of the world economy that is concerned with medicine and health care in the United States. Thus one group of investigators has estimated that by the year 2000 the typical physician will be spending less than one-fourth of his time in the activities comprehended today in the term *direct patient care*. Half the patient visits outside the hospital will be to nonphysicians, one-third of these for services for well people rather than sick patients. Homes will be wired for all kinds of diagnostic and monitoring procedures, the way laboratories and intensive care units are today, it was predicted; some of the services that were seen migrating from hospitals would be concentrated in inexpensive, motel-like parahospitals, or minimedical centers, for ambulatory and convalescing patients.[3]

For another passenger the shape of the future is altogether different. In fact, John G. Freymann, M.D., president of the National Fund for Medical Education, might be looking at the back of the tapestry seen by the year 2000 investigators. Where they saw services migrating from the hospital to homes and minimedical centers, Dr. Freymann's vision has services that were never there before moving into what he has described as the "mission-oriented hospital—a dynamic organization of skilled manpower based on a clear and continuing definition of the health needs of the locality served."[4] There must always be a place in hospitals for the sick, Dr. Freymann believes, but "in this new age our main responsibility has shifted to the vast majority of the population that is well and should be kept that way." The emphasis in the mission-oriented hospital will be on ambulatory services, with a range of facilities matched to a range of problems, from high-technology intensive care to nursing and rehabilitation centers for the aged to motels for the near-well. "Public health services, preventive service, and health education programs will be at the periphery of the complex and coordinated with its many-sided operations, including planning," Dr. Freymann foresees. "No two institutions could be quite the same. There would be room for innumerable organizational arrangements and financial schemes, and no hospital would ever be completed. Continuous feedback of data on the solution of old problems and the appearance of new ones would keep every hospital in dynamic flux and ever ready to adjust to new needs."

While it seems likely that there are many hospital administrators, trustees, and physicians who consider that the flux is already about as dynamic as they can stand and wish it would get less instead of more so, there are oracles for all seasons, and whoever finds the hospital too diminished in one vision of the future and too enriched in another can keep turning to other oracles until he finds one to suit. Thus it is possible to consider that the hospital of the future will be neither denuded of its traditional services nor swollen with new ones but will emerge instead as a cluster of specialized intensive care units, as one authoritative opinion has it, or, in the view of another, that it will be for the most part an ambulatory care center that spins off the greater number of its acutely ill and injured bed patients to a huge, and distant, medical center. It may be an independent, consumer-oriented institution with strong links to the local community or a unit of a consortium or multihospital chain under uniform management, if not absentee ownership. However organized, it may be, as now, a church-owned or community-owned, voluntary, not-for-profit entity, or a profit-making corporation, or a unit of government. It may be financed by patients' fees and insurance, with no more government support than now, or wholly by tax funds with bureaucratic monitoring of every penny of expense. It may still be the dominant force in medical enterprise, or it may have given way to the health maintenance organization, or the health care corporation,* or the medical care foundation,† or some combination or confection composed of parts of all these.

So much divergence of thought suggests that we might do as well in our estimates of the future by turning away from the think tanks and the panels of professional experts who dominate the pages of the journals and the platforms of the meetings and relying instead on tea leaves, or astrology, or storefront metaphysicians with incense and crystal balls. But the fact is that the way we think about what we are doing today and the way we plan, and thus to a large extent the decisions and actions we take, depend on our estimates of what the future will be like, and this is why we keep on straining our eyes at the bewildering domain of possibilities, even when what we see is formidable and frightening, as the ever-moving emptiness of sea or air was to Father Teilhard's nervous passengers.

Even in the bewildering domain of possibilities, however, some seeming certainties emerge. One is that whatever the changes in store for us may be, they will

---

*The health care corporation was the central component of the restructured health care delivery system envisioned in the 1970 report of the American Hospital Association's Special Committee on the Provision of Health Services. The HCC could be either a local government or a private corporation, most likely but not necessarily organized by existing health care providers. It would contract to provide comprehensive health services for a defined population.

†Medical care foundations are nonprofit corporations created by state and county medical societies to offer comprehensive health services, conduct peer review, develop and sponsor health care data systems, and carry on related activities. Initiated in California in the 1950s as a means of providing comprehensive prepaid care under medical sponsorship, the movement grew slowly in California and wasn't active elsewhere until national interest was focused on HMOs and PSROs in the early 1970s. Since then, peer review has become the major activity of the foundations.

come slowly and sequentially, as they have been doing. Here there will be no "Appointed Day" as there was in Great Britain, when on July 5, 1948, all but a handful of the nation's hospitals became the property of the Ministry of Health. Another certainty is that U.S. hospitals will never be all this, or all that, or all anything. Some will become—indeed, some already are—near approximations to Dr. Freymann's mission-oriented hospitals, doing everything for everybody; some will tend to become clusters of intensive care units, and some centers of ambulatory services; some will be joined with others in multiple unit systems, and some remain relatively independent; some will reinforce their community ties by seeking and obtaining local support, and some will rely wholly on private borrowing and public fundings; some will be the movers and managers of HMOs or health care corporations or foundations, and some will be moved and managed by them.

As we have seen, what hospitals become will be determined by forces external to the institution to a greater extent than has been the case in the past, but not wholly. For many years to come, the shape of the hospital's services and structure will be decided largely by its own people, within the restrictions and accommodations demanded by law, regulation, technology, and available resources. The trustees' freedom to decide and act has been diminished, but not destroyed. Whether it is diminished further, and how much, remains also within the power of the trustees themselves to determine, at least in part. It is certainly not true yet, and it may never be true, that there is no proper or important function for the hospital board of trustees as we have known it in the past, as a few government officials and hospital authorities have posited. It can be argued more persuasively that the contrary is closer to the truth: There has never been a greater need, or a greater opportunity, for hospital trustees who are knowledgeable, forceful, imaginative, and courageous.

Leaving as certainties only that there will be many kinds of hospitals offering many kinds of services under many kinds of arrangements, it is possible still to make some observations about the professional and organizational environment with a reasonable expectation of being on or near the mark. Thus, for example, the private practice of medicine, which many observers a few years ago were saying would vanish beneath a wave of HMOs in our time, has proved itself to be a durable and buoyant organism whose instinct for self-preservation has been demonstrated again and again in its ready adaptations to changing circumstance—most recently in the rapid proliferation of medical care foundations, those medical society offshoots that rose to the challenge of HMOs and PSROs and grew faster than either of them. In fact, the genius who thought to give them the name *foundation* may have done more for medical public relations than anybody since St. Luke. *Medical care foundation* emits vibrations of beneficence and concern compounded with stability and independence, notwithstanding that the organization itself, while it may in many instances make a substantive contribution to the accessibility and efficiency of medical services, in others is nothing more than a holding company for whatever it is the doctors don't like but can't avoid, dedicated as much as anything to keeping PSROs from getting out of hand, holding capitation at arm's length, building a fence around local norms and standards, and watching out for symptoms of independent thought on the part of hospital utilization committees. Hospitals that have been saying the *Nunc Dimittis* for private practice and making plans accordingly had better take another look. It is going to be around for a long time; some of the prophets who said in 1972 that the HMO would be the prevailing mode of health care delivery by 1980 are going to have grandchildren who will grow up to be private practitioners. By that time, it can be expected that all the family practice training programs that have been established in the last half dozen years will have made some inroads on what happens, and the young physician may choose primary care instead of neurosurgery, but that is a lot less certain.

As surely as there will be private practice of medicine, however, there will be a changed arrangement of the hospitals in which the physician will receive his training and conduct his practice. Mergers and multiple-unit management systems are reducing the number of single hospital entities, and it seems likely that this movement will have advanced to a considerable degree over the next few years. Where identity has been retained, the independent hospital will have become a participating member in some kind of consortium or regional arrangement for sharing clinical as well as administrative services. The area planning agencies that were designated in late 1975 will be influential, if not decisive, in determining who does what; by so much, the physician's freedom to practice as he pleases, where he pleases, will be limited further in the years to come.

Responses to limitations on the physician's freedom to practice as he wishes are predictable as to content, if not form, regardless of the nature of the restriction. When it was the rising cost of malpractice lawsuits, the doctors in San Francisco declined to work without better protection; when it was utilization review requirements that were considered oppressive, the AMA sued the government —and won first deferment and then modification; when it has been inadequate compensation and working conditions in public hospitals, house staffs have gone on strike in Chicago, New York, and elsewhere; when their own hospitals have imposed restrictive rules, physicians have organized to fight back, as in the case of the Council of Hospital Medical Staffs, which was founded in New Orleans and spread to California in the early 1970s and by 1975 claimed chapters in half the states and a membership of thousands; where the threat has been generalized, as in the case of rising dissatisfaction with the course of events in the profession and the society, doctors have organized themselves as labor unions.

As the pressure increases for conformity to some standards, compliance with some rules, it appears inevitable that all these forms of resistance will grow accordingly. Their success may be uneven, as it has been in the past, but the aggregate effect of the maneuvers unquestionably slows the rate of imposition of controls on physicians. Whether it is a government agency or a hospital board, the rule-making body must pause to consider what the response to its requirements may be.

When restrictive rules have been imposed on hospitals in the past, the disposition has been to seek compromise through negotiation. As regulatory authority has become more severe in its requirements and more dogmatic in its methods in recent years, however, hospitals and their public representatives have also become more aggressive in their response. On occasion, the tactic of resistance has been confrontation, not compromise. "It is time for hospitals to challenge the myriad regulations that would undermine the quality of care for the sake of cost control, and to further intervene aggressively in political and legislative efforts to ensure an adequate and appropriate course of national health policy development," said Hospitals, J.A.H.A., in a report of the Association's annual convention in 1975.[5] AHA president John Alexander McMahon explained the process: "AHA has adopted a community focus, a view that actions should be based on what is best for the hospital and the community served by the hospital," he said in a convention address. "Litigation, the ultimate in ideological confrontation, represents a failure of negotiation. In the past we've been able to work with government, to convince the regulators on many occasions through well-reasoned argument and frank discussion that their so-called 'necessary measures' were in fact counterproductive or punitive to patients. Through cooperation and negotiation, compromise was reached. If anything has become outmoded, I'm afraid it has been the spirit of negotiation and compromise we used to know. It has been replaced on the part of government by unyielding dogmatism." The ultimate problem is the government's desire to control costs, the hospitals' desire to serve patients, and the absence of any forum for rational discussion of their differences, Mr. McMahon said. "We stand ready to discuss the issues," he concluded. "We seek a restoration of that spirit of negotiation and compromise, but let us also serve notice that if government persists in letting dogmatism rule its reponses, we will represent ourselves, and our patients, in the courts."

Whether it was in response to the stiffening resistance of doctors and hospitals to restrictive regulation, or in congruence with President Ford's declared intention to loosen the grip of regulatory authority on business and the economy generally, or simply the change in approach of a new Secretary of HEW, there were signs in late 1975 that the unyielding dogmatism on the part of government might yield a little. In a matter of weeks following the effective date of his appointment, Secretary F. David Mathews had told a congressional subcommittee that he did not intend to enforce withholding of federal Medicaid funds to states that didn't have effective utilization review programs until he had examined the sanctions called for in the law at further length. The existing penalty, he said, seemed "so severe that it has the potential of crippling a state's Medicaid program." In seemingly related moves, the new Secretary consulted with representatives of the AMA and agreed to redraft the controversial utilization review regulations for Medicare and Medicaid patients, and the AMA withdrew its suit seeking a permanent injunction against enforcement of the rules; at the same time, the Secretary agreed to confer with representatives of the Pharmaceutical Manufacturers' Association looking toward resolution of the controversy over the so-called "maximum allowable cost" limitation on payment for drugs in Medicare and Medicaid—another regulation that had been vigorously resisted by doctors and hospitals. With the exception of the utilization review requirement, which had been declared unconstitutional by doctors and unworkable by hospitals, there was no assurance that any of the regulations would be modified substantially, but there was cause for hoping this would be the case and, at least, it was possible to believe there might be a rebirth of the spirit of negotiation and compromise in the offing.

If the early moves by the new Secretary should indeed be harbingers of a new and less combative era in hospital-government relations, it may turn out to be more truce than peace. Setting aside the border incidents that are certain to occur in the application of the rewritten utilization review regulations and the planning law that has yet to be implemented, and the Occupational Safety and Health Act that has not yet made its full impact felt in hospitals, and the Environmental Protection Act, and a few others, the truce might last just as long as the Congress fails to enact another major entitlement that has been under discussion in congressional committees and professional circles intensively for the past five years and episodically for the past 35 years: some form of national health insurance. In 1974, it appeared that a kind of consensus had been reached: There were considered to be millions of Americans whose access to health services was inadequate or nonexistent, and more millions whose scanty health insurance coverage left them exposed to the risk of financial hardship. There would be a national plan—some thought as early as 1975 or 1976—that would include comprehensive benefits for poor and low-income families, coverage of long-term,

high-expense "catastrophic" illness for everybody, and mandated health insurance paid for by employers and employees for the working population. Only the
details remained to be worked out, it was commonly believed.

A year later, there was a lot less certainty that it would happen this way.
Nobody wanted to say there was no need; even the AMA had agreed there was,
but the conviction had lost some of its authority among the urgencies of unemployment and inflation and recession. Nobody was quite as certain, either, that
the proposed plan would make that much difference; for example, it didn't even
touch some of the worst problems, like those of poor people with no knowledge of
or access to any health services, the aged in nursing homes, and long-term
psychiatric patients. While it was reported that the Ford Administration would
introduce a national health insurance bill in 1976, the Administration's freeze on
new spending programs was a countervailing force suggesting that any health
insurance bill considered by the Congress that year would have to be limited in
scope and cost in order to have any chance of enactment. Comprehensive
national health insurance, inevitably to be accompanied by new controls on
utilization and cost, was hull down on the far horizon.

The next thrust of regulation is generally seen as coming from the states'
exercise of authority given the Health Systems Agencies in P.L. 93-641 to allow
or disallow changes in hospital facilities and services, and eventually to review
hospital budgets. As John W. Kauffman, former chairman of the Board of
Trustees of the American Hospital Association, said in Trustee magazine: "An
industry crosses the line between private and public when three elements of
control are present. First, there are controls on so-called market entry. The
hospital field has that in certification-of-need and licensure legislation. Second are
price controls. Hospitals have that through state rate review mechanisms and
other third-party controls on hospital rates. Third, there are controls on quality.
Again, we have licensure; we have medical audit under the Joint Commission on
Accreditation of Hospitals, and we have Professional Standards Review Organizations. In my book, all this makes hospitals a public utility just as much as the gas,
phone, and light companies. The difference is that they have it in writing and we
don't; they can protect themselves and we can't; they will benefit and we won't."[6]
As public utilities, Mr. Kauffman said, hospitals should enjoy public safeguards
such as due process, the opportunity to be heard on government decisions affecting
the industry, and the right to review and appeal regulations. Eventually these
rights will be secured for hospitals as they have been for other utilities, but it takes
time and trial and hardship to develop a system of controls that works. There have
been some hardships already, and there are sure to be more.

Another public policy decision whose impact on hospitals has been rising for the past year but still remains to be borne in the uncertain future was the removal of hospital exemption from provisions of the National Labor Relations Act. The labor lawyer, the negotiator, the organizer, and the arbitrator are becoming familiar figures in hospital corridors, the grievance committee as much a part of the administrative machinery as the planning or audit committee. Of course, these are not new phenomena; in many parts of the country unions and collective bargaining, strikes and threats of strikes, have been around for years, and the economic security program of the American Nurses' Association in many of the jurisdictions has been in effect a union wearing professional clothes—and not therefore any easier to deal with, either. Removal of the exemption was probably inevitable as hospitals became increasingly recognized not just as asylums for the sick and injured but also as a major industry whose millions of employees were a measurable segment of the national work force that could not be considered as separate or different from the mainstream of U.S. labor. Yet the exemption was also in a way recognition of the sanctity of the hospital mission, and its removal was thus an invitation to unions to occupy territory where many had hesitated to advance. They don't hesitate any more. Thus major policy decisions and continuing concerns of hospital boards and management everywhere have another new dimension, beginning with a continuing examination of personnel policies and practices and often ending at the bargaining table. Sometimes the picket line.

Incredibly, it has happened that the conversation on the picket line today may consider not strike benefits and grievances, but, say, the efficacy of the corticosteroids as an alternative to antihistamines in the relief of bronchoconstriction. The doctors' strike, which only yesterday seemed as unthinkable as an infamy of angels, is a reality. Confined for the most part to house staffs seeking not so much increases in pay as relief from intolerable working hours and conditions in chronically underfinanced public hospitals, the doctors' strikes have been rationalized as efforts to improve patient care that deteriorates because of the protested conditions.

This is a reasonable enough proposition, but it nevertheless evades the underlying issue of all work stoppages in the hospital: Patient care may deteriorate to the vanishing point when the people who provide it walk off their jobs. Patient care may also be jeopardized when collective bargaining agreements dilute or interfere with the control exercised by professionals and supervisory personnel, and this is the reason hospitals have always resisted unionization. But unions insist that the sanctity of patient care is a screen behind which hospitals have concealed low wages, onerous working conditions, and unfair labor practices, and this was true enough in enough places to help persuade the Congress that the hospital exemption from the National Labor Relations Act could not be sustained. So now, because some hospitals unquestionably needed to be restrained from engaging in unfair practices, all hospitals must live with the constraints of the law and the inconsistencies and hardships of its application. As Walter Lippmann once wrote, "The problems of democracy often prove to be unmanageable by democratic methods."

This may be true, too, in the case of the decision of the doctors who stopped working in San Francisco hospitals in May 1975 in an effort to bring pressure on the state legislature to act in the malpractice crisis. They got some of the relief they were looking for, and some additional action from the legislature that they hadn't been looking for and that wasn't immediately recognizable as relief, at a cost in losses to the affected hospitals that probably can't be measured and a cost in public esteem that certainly can't be. The doctors in California were suffering hardship, as they are elsewhere in the malpractice contretemps; it is understandable that they should cry out in pain, as they have been doing; and it is possible to sympathize with them in their predicament without applauding their strategy. A lot of remedies are being proposed: self-insurance, and reinsurance pools, and the no-fault system of claims and benefits, and limits on liability and contingent fees, and arbitration boards, and even spreading the malpractice risk by adding the premiums to the consumers' health insurance instead of the providers' liability insurance. Some of the states have passed laws introducing some of these, most notably limits on liability, and some of the professional associations are organizing self-insurance and reinsurance pools, and most of the proposed remedies will be tested sooner or later.

But nobody really knows what will work and what won't, so there isn't going to be any one clear road to salvation. As the report of the President's Commission on Medical Malpractice said a few years ago, the root cause of malpractice liability and malpractice lawsuits is malpractice, and so it may be that the most promising road of all, painfully rocky as it seems at times—and especially, as now, when we are just entering on it—is quality assurance, and we aren't going to find out whether that will work or not right away, either.

Meanwhile, medical societies and hospital associations and insurance companies that have been urging physicians and hospitals to spend more time with their patients and take more pains to explain what they are doing, and why, and what results may reasonably be expected, and what may not, are on the right track. But the track is uphill, because, as we have seen, the physician in today's specialized practice may be a formidable stranger instead of a trusted friend and the hospital a technological nightmare instead of a healing dream. Tender loving care is in the mind of the patient as much as the hands of the physician; its loss is a part of the price we pay for progress. Nobody sued the doctor who made house calls.

The sensitivity of physicians on this whole aspect of patient care was exhibited in a physician's reply to a medical student who protested a request that students wear white coats to patient demonstrations. "The physician's dress should convey to even his most anxious patient a sense of seriousness of purpose that helps to provide reassurance and confidence that his or her complaints will be dealt with competently," he wrote in a communication that was published in the New England Journal of Medicine. [7] "In my opinion, blue jeans, loud shirts without ties, and similar dress are inappropriate, especially when you are dealing with patients who are members of generations older than yours. Casual or slovenly dress is likely to convey, rightly or wrongly, casual or inattentive professional handling of their problem. Such a patient may respond in an inhibited manner, fail to volunteer information, refuse to carry out a recommended diagnostic or management program, fail to keep appointments, and be uncomfortable enough to seek help elsewhere. The rapport so anxiously sought for with your patient may be irretrievably lost."

The physician's communication obviously touched a sensitive nerve, and a subsequent issue of the Journal carried a number of letters:[8] "The patient finds it difficult to establish the necessary relation with and confidence in the medical attendant who looks like and behaves no differently from, if not worse than, his own children," said a physician. "I don't want my doctor to be my pal, my big brother or a rap partner," said a patient, "I can get that elsewhere. A certain discipline and a certain regard for the niceties of civilized behavior are necessary adjuncts of professionalism." Another correspondent reported a study of outpatients in New York and San Francisco in which 96 percent of 560 patients in the sample "had a visual image of the typical doctor as a white, clean-shaven, short-haired man between 30 and 50 years old conservatively dressed in a white coat." A pathologist insisted that dress is important in the laboratory. "How would you feel being approached for an intravenous sample by a technologist wearing dungarees and a sweatshirt?" he wanted to know.

Not everybody agreed. A physician at one medical school said it depended on the patient; Spanish-speaking patients want a physician who speaks Spanish and don't care what he has on. Another argued that dignity has been overrated. "The aloofness and detachment of many members of the profession is wrapped in the cloak of dignity," he said. "It is from this stance that doctors, nurses, and receptionists peer across an ever-widening gulf to view our patients. This is not to imply that we need to be buddies with everyone who seeks our help. We must continue to touch our patients. Touch is a variation of a modicum of healing. Judgment, common sense, and touch. A tremendous amount of stress can be lifted from our lives if we would simply be what we started out to be back in college: sympathetic people, working to help distressed patients, honestly, courageously, daily—and to hell with dignity."

Finally, 75 medical students at Stanford, where the argument about white coats started, signed a manifesto: "If the student physician's communication of his or her seriousness of purpose is held to depend on attire, a certain percentage of patients will be lost to us no matter how we dress. Instead of simply giving up on these patients, we would prefer to win their trust through a caring attitude, in spite of any preconceptions that they might have about what our appearance should be. Dr. Kriss finds it disrespectful for students to dress inappropriately during a patient demonstration. Since we have shown that we disagree with his view of what is appropriate dress, we believe that if respect is to be mutual and based on trust, it must include a willingness on his part to trust us to make our own decisions about how we present ourselves to patients. We as students are genuinely concerned with improving the quality of our relations with patients, faculty, and other members of the health care team. We cannot improve these relations without changing them somewhat. We hope that these changes can be accomplished in the spirit of mutual trust and respect."

The spirited criticism and impassioned defense of white coats might be considered an absurdity if it didn't suggest an awareness that something that is more than jacket-deep is going wrong with the doctor-patient relationship and the practice of medicine. Something is, and thoughtful critics inside and outside the profession have been concerned to describe and analyze it and start looking for answers. The most Draconian of the critics is Ivan Illich, the educator and former priest whose view is that by "industrializing" medicine and, as he says, "medicalizing" society, we are dehumanizing patients and robbing them of the will and ability to cope for themselves. According to Mr. Illich, modern medicine "assumes that all the ills of everyone ought to be treated, whatever the predictable outcome. Unfortunately, this therapeutic mania is infectious and has crippled the traditional art of sick care."[9] Mr. Illich's proposed remedy is reminiscent of the solution he suggested a few years ago for the problems of the public school system: abolish it. "The true miracle of modern medicine is diabolical," he says now. "It consists of making not only individuals but whole populations survive on inhumanly low levels of personal health. By refusing medicine, each one can question the social base of industrial society at that point at which it is most intimately entrenched."

Mr. Illich is not all invective. His strictures are documented with references to reports in the medical literature of indiscriminate medication, unnecessary surgery, doubtful results of high-technology support systems, and similar excesses that worry thoughtful physicians everywhere. One of them, Professor D. W.

Harding of London University, called Mr. Illich's book "an effective polemical expression of the diffuse dissatisfaction with medicine which has been gathering force for the last decade or so."[10]

Ivan Illich is not alone in calling for revolution, not just reform. Another critic whose recommendations add up to dissolution of the medical care system is Rick J. Carlson, a lawyer who has done research in medical care at Interstudy, the health services research center in Minneapolis, and is now a consultant to the Institute of Medicine, National Academy of Sciences, and adjunct assistant professor of medicine at Boston University School of Medicine. "With the exception of a few hardy rural practitioners and family physicians, medicine has compartmentalized the body into finer and finer machine parts," Mr. Carlson said.[11] "It is one thing to treat a patient as a machine, ignoring a rich store of information that is related to health and functioning, and yet another to further subdivide the machine into its constituent parts. In the former medicine, at least the possibility existed for holistic treatment. In today's medicine the task is nearly impossible." The whole medical care system has less impact on health than social and environmental factors have, according to Mr. Carlson. "We must start over in our efforts to achieve health," he concluded. "This will require new thinking and new approaches, and it will also require abandoning much of the system that now provides medical care."

Now it is not likely that people in large numbers are going to follow Mr. Illich and start refusing all treatment, preferring pain to palliative, or that either physicians or politicians will consider that Mr. Carlson has the right answer and start dismembering the system, boarding up hospitals and turning medical schools into factories. But many of the new initiatives in medicine arise from the cognate belief that there must come a turning away from the value system that has pushed specialization and technology beyond the point where humaneness can accompany them. The new family practice training programs, the new departments of social medicine and community medicine at the medical schools and hospitals, the new programs in holistic medicine and humanistic medicine, the emphasis on primary care at the medical schools and ambulatory care at the hospitals, the push for research in effective methods of teaching people how to take better care of themselves—all these are attempts to redress the imbalance that has become apparent as we keep on pushing more and more money and manpower and machinery into medical care and get back less and less improvement in the health status of the population.

It is possible to believe, and many hospital trustees and administrators and physicians do believe, that the surge of interest in the noninstitutional, nontechnical, nonspecialized, nonprofessional aspects of health care represents a threat to hospitals, whose proper business is to take care of the acutely ill and seriously injured and let somebody else worry about these lesser concerns that have always been on the outskirts of medical interest and ought to remain there. It is possible to believe this, but it isn't necessary, because it is also possible to believe that the proper interest of hospitals and physicians is health, and so whatever contributes to health is the proper business of hospitals and physicians. For as long as hospital boards of trustees are free to decide what the missions of their institutions shall be, and the view here is that this will be for generations to come, trustees who see the business of the hospital as acute care will govern institutions that are essentially clusters of intensive care units, islands of technique in larger systems of health care. Trustees who see the business of the hospital as health will govern the larger systems.

REFERENCES

Chapter 2

1. Fishbein, M. A History of the American Medical Association, 1847 to 1947. Philadelphia: W. B. Saunders Co., 1947, p. 398.
2. Darling v. Charleston Memorial Hospital, 211 N.E. 2d 253 (Ill. 1965).

Chapter 3

1. Porter, K. W. A profile of the hospital trustee. Trustee. 28:21, Jan. 1975. This is a condensed report of a comprehensive survey conducted for the American Hospital Association magazine Trustee. References to unpublished findings of the survey appear elsewhere in this report.
2. MacEachern, M. T. Hospital Organization and Management. 2nd ed. Chicago: Physicians' Record Co., 1946, pp. 73-84.
3. Nelson, R. A. The Governance of Voluntary Teaching Hospitals in New York City. New York City: The Josiah Macy Jr. Foundation, 1974, pp. 27-28.
4. Hospital Care in the United States, Report of the Commission on Hospital Care. New York City: Commonwealth Fund, 1947.
5. Stern v. Lucy Webb Hayes National Training School for Deaconesses and Missionaries, 367 F. Supp. 536 (D.C., D.C. Nov. 30, 1973); 381 F. Supp. 1003 (D.C., D.C. 1974).
6. Comptroller General of the United States. Report to the Congress: A Proposal for Disclosure of Contractual and Financial Arrangements Between Hospitals and Members of Their Governing Boards and Hospitals and Their Medical Specialists. Washington, DC: U.S. General Accounting Office, Apr. 1975.
7. Ibid. Appendixes II, III, and IV.
8. Barr, J. W. Address to the Western Regional Meeting of the Bank Administration Institute, Los Angeles, Mar. 26, 1973.
9. Survey for Trustee (chapter 3, note 1).
10. Survey for Trustee (chapter 3, note 1).

11. Underwood, J. M. A trustee looks at positive and negative trusteeship. *Trustee*. 26:1, Mar. 1973.
12. Catholic Hospital Association. *Guidelines on the Responsibilities, Functions, and Selection Criteria for Hospital Boards of Trustees* (revised). St. Louis: CHA, 1974.

Chapter 4

1. Survey for *Trustee* (chapter 3, note 1).
2. Coblentz, W. K. A Trustee's Dilemma. Address to a joint seminar of the American College of Hospital Administrators and the Academy of Hospital Public Relations, San Diego, May 29, 1975.

Chapter 5

1. Fuchs, V. R. *Who Shall Live?* New York City: Basic Books, Inc., 1975.
2. Nelson, op. cit. (chapter 3, note 3).
3. American Hospital Association. *Management Review Program. Hospital Governing Board.* Chicago: AHA, 1971, pp. 5-6.
4. Nelson, op. cit. (chapter 3, note 3).
5. Commission on Education for Health Administration. *Education for Health Administration*, vol. 1. Ann Arbor, MI: Health Administration Press, 1975, p. 15.

Chapter 6

1. *Darling v. Charleston Community Hospital*, 211 N.E. 2d 253 (Ill. 1965).
2. *Gonzales v. Nork and Mercy Hospitals of Sacramento, Cal.* Super. Ct., No. 228-566, Sacramento County (Nov. 1973).
3. Porterfield, J. D. Comments from the director. *Perspectives on Accreditation.* 1:1, Jan.-Feb. 1975.
4. Related to the author by the AHA representative.
5. Slee, V.N. Address to the Hospital Medical Staff Conference conducted by the Estes Park Institute, Sun Valley, ID, May 1975.
6. Illich, I. *Medical Nemesis: The Expropriation of Health.* London: Calder and Boyars, Ltd., 1974.
7. Reported in Noie, N. Gearing up for PSROs—did anyone say it would be easy? *The Hospital Medical Staff.* 4:26, Feb. 1975.

8. Cunningham, J. D. The hospital-physician relationship: hospital responsibility for malpractice of physicians. *Washington Law Review.* 50:385, Feb. 1975.
9. Rubsamen, D. S. Even more legal controls on the physician's hospital practice. *New England Journal of Medicine.* 292:917, Apr. 24, 1975.
10. *Moore v. Board of Carson-Tahoe Hospital,* 495 P 2d 605 (1972).
11. *Purcell v. Zimbelman,* 500 P 2d 335 (1972).
12. Brown, M. B. Trustee Involvement on Medical Staff Committees, draft, June 1975.
13. American College of Hospital Administrators Task Force, Recommendations on Standards to the Joint Commission on Accreditation of Hospitals, Adopted by the Board of Governors, May 24, 1974.
14. Catholic Hospital Association. *Guidelines on Roles and Relationships of Board, Chief Executive Officer, and Medical Staff of Catholic Hospital and Long-Term Care Facilities.* St. Louis: CHA, 1974.
15. Donnelly, P. R. Address to the Hospital Medical Staff Conference conducted by the Estes Park Institute, Sun Valley, ID, May 1975.
16. American Hospital Association. *Governance of Health Care Institutions.* Chicago: AHA, 1974.
17. McMahon, J. A. Hospital-physician relations: where do we go from here? *Trustee.* 28:25, Mar. 1975.

Chapter 7

1. *New York Times*, June 15, 1975.
2. Hinderer, H. Financing toward Bankruptcy. Address to the Colorado Hospital Association, Oct. 4, 1974. Published in *Hospital Financial Management.* 29:10, Nov. 1975.
3. Altman, S. H. Informal conference with a group of visiting hospital representatives.
4. Workshop session at the annual convention, American Nursing Home Association, 1972.
5. American Hospital Association. *Guidelines for Review and Approval of Rates for Health Care Institutions and Services by a State Commission,* accepted by the Board of Trustees, Feb. 9, 1972.
6. Scroggins, R. E. Hospital costs: a joint trustee-administrator-physician responsibil-

ity. *Trustee.* 28:19, Aug. 1972.

7. Garrett, R. What the SEC Expects of Corporate Directors. Address to a corporate directors conference sponsored by Arthur D. Little, Inc., Washington, DC, Dec. 17, 1974.

8. Barr, J. W. The Role of the Professional Director. Address at a seminar at Loyola College, Baltimore, Apr. 8, 1975.

9. What's your opinion? *Trustee.* 28:36, May 1975.

10. American Association of Fund-Raising Counsel, annual report, 1974.

11. Blendon, R. J. The changing role of private philanthropy in health affairs. *New England Journal of Medicine.* 292:946, May 1, 1975.

12. Haney, W. R., and Haney, C. A. III. Periodic campaigns overcome donor shifts. *Hospitals, J.A.H.A.* 49:57, June 1, 1975.

13. Filer, J. H., quoted in Kernaghan, S. G., and Manzano, A. The changing face of philanthropy. *Trustee.* 28:17, June 1975.

Chapter 8

1. Bicknell, W. J., and Walsh, D. C. Certification of need: the Massachusetts experience. *New England Journal of Medicine.* 292:1054, May 15, 1975.

2. Nelson, op. cit., Appendix A (chapter 3, note 3).

3. Green, H. A. Long-range planning in realistic steps. *Trustee.* 26:25, May 1973.

Chapter 9

1. Brown, R. E. *Conversations: The Evolving Role of the Hospital Trustee.* Philadelphia: ARA Hospital Food Management, 1969, p. 13.

2. Related by Hans Mauksch, Department of Sociology, University of Missouri, Columbia.

3. *Medical Malpractice: Report of the Secretary's Commission on Medical Malpractice.* Washington, DC: Department of Health, Education, and Welfare, 1973.

4. Fuchs, op. cit. (chapter 5, note 1).

5. Sidel, V. W. Quality for Whom? Effects of Professional Responsibility for Quality of Health Care on Equity. Address to the 1975 Annual Health Conference of the New York Academy of Medicine, Apr. 24-25, 1975.

Chapter 10

1. Grapski, L. F. *Conversations: Redefining the Role of the Hospital Trustee.* Philadelphia: ARA Hospital Food Management, 1974, pp. 20-21.

2. Trustee training program produces active, responsible board members. *Cross-Reference.* 5:1, May 1975.

3. Greenleaf, R. K. *Trustees as Servants.* Cambridge, MA: Center for Applied Studies, 1974, pp. 22-23.

4. Survey for *Trustee* (chapter 3, note 1).

5. Nelson, op. cit. (chapter 3, note 3).

6. Schechter, D. S. *Agenda for Continuing Education: A Challenge to Health Care Institutions.* Chicago: Hospital Research and Educational Trust, 1974, p. 61.

7. Stark, N. Quoted in Schechter (note 6).

8. Barzun, J. *Teacher in America.* Garden City, NY: Doubleday Anchor Books, 1954, p. 67.

9. Quoted in Barzun (note 8).

Chapter 11

1. Meadows, D. L., and others. *Limits to Growth: A Report for the Club of Rome Project on the Predicament of Mankind.* New York City: Universe Books, 1972.

2. Oltmans, W. L., editor. *On Growth: The Crisis of Exploding Population and Resource Depletion.* New York City: Capricorn Books, G. P. Putnam's Sons, 1974.

3. Bender, A. D., and others. Delphic study examines developments in medicine. *Futures.* June 1969.

4. Freymann, J. G. *The American Health Care System: Its Genesis and Trajectory.* New York City: Medcom, Inc., 1974, p. 385.

5. The 1975 annual convention in review. *Hospitals, J.A.H.A.* 49:67, Sept. 1, 1975.

6. Kauffman, J. W. Are hospitals becoming public utilities? *Trustee.* 28:24, Aug. 1975.

7. Kriss, J. P. On white coats and other matters. *New England Journal of Medicine.* 292:1024, May 8, 1975.

8. Coats, white or soiled. *New England Journal of Medicine.* 292:563, Sept. 11, 1975.

9. Illich, op. cit. (chapter 6, note 6).

10. Harding, D. W. Home remedies. *New York Review of Books.* 22:5, Apr. 17, 1975.

11. Carlson, R. J. *The End of Medicine.* New York City: John Wiley & Sons, Inc., 1975.

INDEX

Accountability of governing board
  effect on trustee performance, iv
  impact of external factors, iv
Accountability of trustees
  current trends, 31-33
  for quality of medical service, 31-32
  response to the press and broadcast media, 31
  traditional, 30-31
Accreditation standards for hospitals, 27
ACHA. See American College of Hospital Administrators
Administrative authority, precedence over medical staff authority, 91-92
Administrative office, organization, 146
Administrative Procedure Act, 14
Administrator
  accountable to governing board, 48
  accountability to governing authority, 89-92
  as agent with delegated authority, 47-48
  as agent of governing board, 90
  appointed by board of trustees, 58
  in church-affiliated hospitals, 88
  as coordinator of all hospital groups, 91-92
  educational seminars for, 142-44
  executive growth and selection, 146
  executive recruitment, 61
  as member of governing board, 47-48
  modern role, 88-92
  personal and professional qualifications, 66-67
  position and function, 87-92
  qualifications, 61
  recruitment from within, 70-71
  responsibilities and duties, 67-68, 89
  selection, 146
  special skills needed, 92
  as subordinate to governing board and medical staff, 88
  as super board member, 52
  task summarized, 68-69
  traditional contrasted with modern, ii
  traditional role, 87-88
Allegheny General Hospital, 142
Altman, Stuart H., 96-97, 101-102
American College of Hospital Administrators (ACHA), 89, 91
American College of Physicians, 26, 62
American College of Surgeons, vi, 25n., 26-27, 32, 35, 62, 73
American Health Facilities, Inc., 121
American Hospital Association, 26, 32, 36, 41, 42, 46, 50, 51, 62, 67, 75, 76, 86, 91, 96, 97, 98, 100, 101, 116, 118, 124, 130, 131, 132, 147, 156, 158
American Hospital Association House of Delegates, 36

American Medical Association, 26, 36, 42, 78, 155, 157
American Nurses' Association, 159
American Security and Trust Company, 43
Annual report, purposes of, i, 132-33

Babcock, Kenneth, 74
Bankers
  as choices for trusteeship, 34
  representation on governing boards, 39-44
Bargielski, Leo, 143
Barr, Joseph H., 43, 105-106, 107
Barzun, Jacques, 150
Bicknell, William J., 113, 122-23
"Bitching level," as management performance standard, 63
Blendon, Robert J., 108-109
Blue Cross, i, vii, 24, 25n., 29, 95, 97, 100, 101, 108, 115, 121. See also Blue Cross-Blue Shield; Plan for Hospital Care
Blue Cross Association, 76
Blue Cross-Blue Shield, 121
Board. See Board of directors; Board of trustees; Governing board
Board of directors. See also Board of trustees; Governing board
  typical executive committee meetings described, 1-12
Board of trustees. See also Executive committee; Governing board; Super board; Trustees
  change in accountability, iv
  committee effectiveness, 54-56
  committee responsibilities, 54-56
  committee structure, 54-56
  communication with medical staff, 36
  defending cost data, 118
  delegation of authority to administrator, 90-91
  educational seminars for, 142-44
  essential functions, 58
  future function, 154
  members as super trustees, 51-53
  need for information, 146-47
  "package of reserved powers," 90-91
  physician members, 85-86
  planning committee, 121-23
  policies for crisis situations, 56-57
  as policymaker, 56-58
  related to administration, 56
  responsibilities, 57-58
  responsibilities and functions, listed, 50
  responsibility for accounting, budget planning, and reporting, 103
  responsibility increasing, 49
  responsibility for long-range planning, 121-23
  responsibility for professional service, 91-92

Plan for Hospital Care, i, iii. *See also* Blue Cross
Plan Utilization Review (PUR), 76
Porterfield, John D., 74, 76, 77
Prepaid group practice
  based in hospitals, 119
  value of, 120-21
Prepaid health plans, 121
Prepayment concept. *See also* Plan for Hospital
    Care
  response to, ii
  seen as socialized medicine, ii-iii
President. *See* Administrator, as member of gov-
    erning board
President's Commission on Medical Malprac-
    tice, 126, 160
Press, demands on hospital officials, 31
Press and broadcast media, critical of hospitals,
    126-27
A Primer for Hospital Trustees, 149
Private medical practice, future status, 154-55
Professional Activities Study-Medical Audit
    Program, 84
Professional Standards Review Organization
    (PSRO), 24, 117, 141, 154, 158
  as quality assurance agency, 77-79
  related to costs of Medicare and Medicaid,
    77-79
  resistance from physicians, 79-80
Property owners, as choices for trusteeship,
    34-35
PSRO. *See* Professional Standards Review Or-
    ganization
Public relations
  broadened scope, 125-26
  complexity, 125
  contemporary trend, 125
  function, 128
  in fund raising, 133
  importance, 124
  information policy, 128-30
  limited scope, 132-33
  press criticism, 126-27
  responsibility for community involvement,
    138
  specific goals, 132-33
  trustee responsibility, 126
Public representatives, bargaining for health ser-
    vices, 29
PUR. *See* Plan Utilization Review

QAM. *See* Quality Assurance Monitor
QAP. *See* Quality Assurance Program for Medi-
    cal Care in the Hospital
Quality assurance. *See* Medical care, quality as-
    surance

Quality Assurance Monitor (QAM), 76
Quality Assurance Program for Medical Care in
    the Hospital, 79, 84, 87
Quality of medical care. *See* Medical care, evalu-
    ation of quality

Rate review commission. *See also* Rate setting
    commission
  established by states, 100-103
  state vs. federal authority, 102
Rate setting commission, 94-95, 100
Ratio of charges to charges according to cost, iii
Ravdin, I. S., 25n.
RCCAC. *See* Ratio of charges to charges accord-
    ing to cost
"Reasonable cost" reimbursement, in financial
    operations, iii
Regionalization of service, development, 120
Regional Medical Programs
  planning and service functions, 27-28
  resistance to, 27-28
Reimbursement contracts, related to financial
    condition, 108
Reporting of medical results, demand for, 83-85
Robert Wood Johnson Foundation, 108
Robinson, Don, 74
Rockefeller Foundation, 67
Roentgen, Wilhelm, 23
Rubsamen, David S., 81, 82
Russell, Bertrand, vii

Sacred Heart Hospital, 25n.
San Francisco hospitals, exodus of anesthesiol-
    ogists, 56, 61
Schechter, Daniel S., 147-49
Scroggins, Raymond E., 103, 104
SEC. *See* U.S. Securities and Exchange Com-
    mission
Secretary's Advisory Committee on Hospital Ef-
    fectiveness, 120
Selection of trustees
  lowering of barriers to physicians, 35-37
  occupational and status factors, 34-35
  traditional mode, 34-35
Shared services, 95, 112-13
Sidel, Victor W., 137-38
Smith, Francis, 25n.
Social Security Act, 26, 42
Social Security Administration. *See* U.S. Social
    Security Administration
Social Security Amendments of 1965, 26
Social Security Amendments of 1972, 28, 77,
    120
Southwestern Michigan Hospital Council, 62
Specialism. *See* Medical specialization